Maynooth
College
reflects on
COVID-19

New Realities
in Uncertain Times

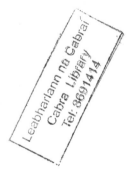

Published by Messenger Publications, 2021

ISBN 9781788123327

Cover collage from photograph © Paul Shuang / Shutterstock
Designed by Messenger Publications Design Department
Typeset in Adobe Caslon Pro, Adminster & Cancelleresca Script
Printed by Johnswood Press Limited

Messenger Publications,
37 Leeson Place, Dublin D02 E5V0
www.messenger.ie

Maynooth College Reflects on COVID-19

New Realities in Uncertain Times

Edited by

Jeremy Corley, Neil Xavier O'Donoghue & Salvador Ryan
Foreword by Archbishop Eamon Martin

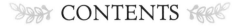 CONTENTS

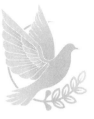

Foreword

Archbishop Eamon Martin

*A*nyone watching Pope Francis on Friday, 27 March 2020, standing in stark solitude in an empty St Peter's Square, could hardly fail to have been moved by the sight of this lone figure in white delivering his *Urbi et Orbi* message. Reflecting on the story of Jesus' stilling of the storm that frightened his disciples (Mk 4:35–41), the Pope spoke in a prophetic way:

> 'Why are you afraid? Have you no faith?' Lord, your word this evening strikes us and concerns us, all of us. In this world, that you love more than we do, we have gone ahead at breakneck speed, feeling powerful and able to do anything. Greedy for profit, we let ourselves get caught up in things, and lured away by haste. We did not stop at your reproach to us, we were not shaken awake by wars or injustice across the world, nor did we listen to the cry of the poor or of our ailing planet. We carried on regardless, thinking we would stay healthy in a world that was sick. Now that we are in a stormy sea, we implore you: 'Wake up, Lord!'[1]

---

1   Pope Francis, *Urbi et Orbi* message, 27 March 2020. Online, http://www.vatican.va/content/francesco/en/homilies/2020/documents/papa-francesco_20200327_omelia-epidemia.html.

Later in this message, Pope Francis called us to re-evaluate our lives and develop a deeper trust in God:

> Faith begins when we realise we are in need of salvation. We are not self-sufficient. By ourselves we founder. We need the Lord, like ancient navigators needed the stars. Let us invite Jesus into the boats of our lives. Let us hand over our fears to him, so that he can conquer them. Like the disciples, we will experience that with him on board there will be no shipwreck. Because this is God's strength: turning to the good everything that happens to us, even the bad things. He brings serenity into our storms, because with God life never dies.

In August 2020, the Pontifical Council for Interreligious Dialogue and the World Council of Churches released a joint document, calling on Christians to develop a sense of interreligious solidarity to confront the COVID-19 crisis.[2] The document eloquently describes our recent experience:

> The COVID-19 pandemic has had an impact on the global community with unavoidable immediacy and with little preparedness on our part. It has dramatically altered everyone's daily life, and powerfully exposed the vulnerability that all humans share. Alongside the millions who have been infected physically, many more have been affected psychologically, economically, politically and religiously; all have been deprived of public worship. People have struggled to cope with death and grief, especially with the inability to be with their loved ones at their deathbeds and perform their last rites and funerals in a

---

2   The Pontifical Council for Interreligious Dialogue (PCID) and the World Council of Churches (WCC), *Serving a Wounded World in Interreligious Solidarity: A Christian Call to Reflection and Action During COVID-19* (Geneva: WCC / Vatican City: PCID, 2020).

dignified manner. The lockdown has brought the world economy to its knees, and global hunger could double, due to this catastrophe. It has also contributed to an increase in domestic violence. The requirements of physical and social distancing have meant isolation for many people. Despair, anxiety and insecurity have come to dominate human lives. The coronavirus has affected all – rich and poor, the elderly and children, persons in cities and villages, farmers and industrialists, workers and students.[3]

During this time of COVID-19 restrictions, for instance, the elderly have been disproportionately impacted. The virus has wreaked havoc in nursing homes where stringent restrictions on visiting have added to a sense of isolation and vulnerability. Many grand-parents have been missing the physical company and affection of their grandchildren – especially their hugs! The effect of the pandemic on older members of society has been highlighted by Pope Francis in his October 2020 encyclical letter, *Fratelli Tutti* (FT). He notes that often in modern society, the elderly have been relegated to a sad and lonely existence, because our individual concerns are the only thing that matter to us. He comments:

> We have seen what happened with the elderly in certain places in our world as a result of the coronavirus. They did not have to die that way. Yet something similar had long been occurring during heatwaves and in other situations: older people found themselves cruelly abandoned. We fail to realise that, by isolating the elderly and leaving them in the care of others without the closeness and concern of family members, we disfigure and impoverish the family itself. (FT, 19)

Older people are not the only group in society to have suffered. These past months have been challenging also for young people – I

3   Ibid., 6.

think especially of those for whom 2020 was to have been an important 'graduation' year – from primary school to post-primary; from school to college; from college into the world of work; from engagement to marriage. For them, the joyful celebration of these special transition moments has been cruelly interrupted.

Although public health authorities have understandably focused on the physical health of the population, arguably less attention has been given to promoting people's mental and spiritual health. People with underlying addictions have struggled to maintain recovery. Relationships have been put under pressure. Domestic violence and coercive control situations have been exacerbated. The limitations on social gatherings have added to a sense of loneliness and isolation among many, while the restrictions on funeral gatherings have prevented families and communities from fully expressing and sharing their grief. Moreover, with the closing-down of public worship for months, many people of faith have felt deprived of the spiritual comfort and solidarity that gathering in prayer and praise can bring during difficult times.

While the pandemic has posed problems for us as individuals, it has also brought great challenges to governments across the globe. In *Fratelli Tutti*, Pope Francis observed the world struggling to grapple with the pandemic: 'For all our hyper-connectivity, we witnessed a fragmentation that made it more difficult to resolve problems that affect us all…. It is my desire that, in this our time, by acknowledging the dignity of each human person, we can contribute to the rebirth of a universal aspiration to fraternity' (FT, 7–8). Later in *Fratelli Tutti*, Pope Francis adds:

> If everything is connected, it is hard to imagine that this global disaster is unrelated to our way of approaching reality, our claim to be absolute masters of our own lives and of all that exists. I do not want to speak of divine retribution, nor would it be sufficient to say that the harm we do to nature is itself the punishment for our offences. The world

is itself crying out in rebellion. We are reminded of the well-known verse of the poet Virgil that evokes the 'tears of things,' the misfortunes of life and history. (FT, 34)

Besides underlining our interconnectedness around the world, this time of global pandemic is also reminding us of our fragility, our shared vulnerability and common need for compassion and love, as well as the hope that faith in God can bring. The Pope has spoken so powerfully of the message of love that is at the heart of the Gospel – a love which reaches out to all of our 'brothers and sisters' who share our common humanity. The witness of so many Christians and others of goodwill who have immersed themselves in mission and outreach to the vulnerable during the pandemic has been inspirational – bringing light into darkness, hope into despair.

Reflecting during the almost surreal Lent and Holy Week lockdown of 2020, I likened the journey through the pandemic to a modern day 'Way of the Cross'. There have been countless 'Veronicas' and 'Simons': amazing health workers and carers who have put themselves out to wipe the brow and dry the tears of our suffering brothers and sisters, volunteers carrying groceries, foodstuffs and essentials to those living on their own and so many others who have been sending messages of love, hope and encouragement. These 'Veronicas' and 'Simons' have reminded people that they are not forgotten, and that even if we cannot hold their hands or give them a hug, we hold them closer than before in our hearts. We rightly applaud and publicly acknowledge those who have been keeping essential services going, by denying themselves and taking risks in the cause of compassion, charity and love.

At a personal level, we have learned that every time we say 'no' to going out, make a simple sacrifice or practise self-denial, we are helping to protect health, save lives and contribute to the common good. Where charity and love are found, God is there.

In *Fratelli Tutti* Pope Francis makes a special appeal in the name of justice and mercy for the orphan, the poor, the stranger, the migrant, the refugee and all those on the margins or peripheries of life and society. He envisages an open world motivated by what he calls 'social friendship' and sincere hospitality towards others. I find it particularly challenging when he mentions that, 'Some peripheries are close to us, in the city centres or in our families.' This reminds us here in Ireland to consider who might be left out. We can ask: who do we tend to shuffle over into the margins of society and perhaps try to forget? I sometimes wonder about the impact on us of seeing a homeless person lying on our streets, or of watching live images of thousands of refugees huddled in camps or starving children swatting away flies from their faces – how easily can we shift our gaze, feel sorry for them but never really question our own values, lifestyle, attitudes? This dilemma is at the heart of *Fratelli Tutti*.

These days we hear a lot about 'social distancing'. Perhaps the real social distancing is the way that the great majority of us can get on with our lives seemingly oblivious or 'anaesthetised' to the tremendous suffering, inequality and neglect around us. Solidarity with the poor and vulnerable, Pope Francis says, means looking into their faces, sensing their closeness and trying to help them. It never tolerates any assault on human life or the human dignity of any person. We are called to have a 'gaze transformed by charity' which touches our hearts like the Good Samaritan and shows a preferential love to those in greatest need. At this time of global pandemic, Pope Francis calls us to love each other as God loves us by living the parable of the Good Samaritan every minute of every day. Our civilisation is not omnipotent, so we need to respect the innate dignity of one another – from family to stranger – with love and practical support, so that the human race can flourish.

What the world has been going through these past months will surely be spoken about for a long time. When people look back on 2020–2021, they will tell the story of how the world had to pause; most travel was suspended; people had to isolate themselves from one another and learn new ways to study, to communicate and do business. They will speak of how new opportunities were found for people to gather virtually – not only for lessons, socialising and decision-making – but also for prayer and the praise of God.

When we come to tell the story of COVID-19, I hope we will speak about what we learned during the pandemic: how it made us question our priorities and values; how people were prepared to make sacrifices for the common good and for the protection of health and life; how we came to appreciate those who care for the elderly and the sick, and how charity and heroism can flourish in the midst of crisis. Perhaps we will conclude that 2020 was the year we learned to truly value our friends, family and Church more, because we had to spend so much time apart.

These days of pandemic are inspiring many people to reflect more on their personal life story and faith journey. The pandemic offers an opportunity for a new beginning. We might, for example, consider the impact of the COVID-19 restrictions on our personal lives and values – has it made us more determined to live better and more purposeful lives? Have we become more sensitised to the needs of the vulnerable; more in touch with our own physical, emotional, mental and spiritual needs; more aware of the fragility of our lives, our dependence on one another and on our need for God?

In May 2020, I appealed to theologians and philosophers: 'I hope that philosophers, sociologists and media commentators of Ireland might begin to reflect on and critique how key societal relationships and partnerships have been impacted – for better or worse – by the pandemic. I encourage our theologians to consider what this crisis is saying to us about Church, about our identity and mission, about our relationship with the State, and about how prayer and faith can help sustain believers in a time of anxiety and crisis.'[4] I note that in recent months various insightful and challenging reflections on COVID-19 have been published in magazines and journals.[5]

---

4   Archbishop Eamon Martin, *Homily for Ascension Sunday / World Communications Day*, 25 May 2020.

5   See, for instance, Michael Neary, 'Covid-19 – A Challenge to Faith', *The Furrow* 71 (September 2020): 455–458; Brendan Leahy, 'Ten Covid-19 "Outcomes" for the Church', *The Furrow* 71 (May 2020): 285–291.

Moreover, several Maynooth faculty members contributed useful articles that were published on diocesan websites and also in *Intercom*.

The present volume offers varied responses to my appeal, provided by members and associates of the theology and philosophy faculties of St Patrick's College, Maynooth. I hope that Catholics, lay and ordained, will take up this book and ponder its contents, and that priests, religious and parish groups, even those meeting online, will find it a helpful springboard for discussion and reflection.

In a similar way I encourage as many people as possible to capture in poetry, prose, music or art what the pandemic has been saying to us – about Church and society, about identity and mission, about power and vulnerability, about suffering and mortality, about charity, faith and hope.

One day all these stories, memories and reflections will help to form the narrative that future generations will study to understand how the world and its people coped in challenging times.

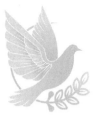

Introduction

*Jeremy Corley, Neil Xavier O'Donoghue
and Salvador Ryan*

*W*here has God been in the midst of COVID-19? The pandemic has turned our lives upside-down in so many ways. The media has repeatedly reported on medical and social aspects – the effects on hospitals and care homes, schools and colleges, businesses and workplaces. Religious implications have often focused on the transfer of Masses to online platforms, and the postponements of events like Holy Communions, Confirmations and weddings. But the effect of COVID-19 is far broader and deeper. While the gradual rollout of the vaccine has given grounds for hope, the months of pandemic have caused profound changes in Church and society, deserving careful reflection.

Key insights appear in the conversations of Pope Francis with Austen Ivereigh, published in December 2020.[1] The volume, entitled *Let Us Dream: The Path to a Better Future*, was written by the Pope in response to COVID-19. In his answers to the interview questions, he indicates how the pandemic has provided an opportunity for us all to slow down, take stock, and design better ways of living together on this earth. According to Pope Francis, this crisis is a threshold moment, when God is entering our history, even in these times of

---

1   Pope Francis in Conversation with Austen Ivereigh, *Let Us Dream: The Path to a Better Future* (London: Simon & Schuster UK, 2020).

suffering and crisis. We are challenged personally to open ourselves to God in order to receive the Spirit who leads us in a new direction, both in our individual lives and in society.

Pope Francis believes that our merciful God is holding out graces to us in our time of tribulation, but if we close ourselves off, we will miss them. Now God is offering us a choice about the direction of our future, a choice between changing or refusing to do so. The Pope suggests that if we understand where the Spirit is calling us, we will make the right choices. But there is a need for prayer, reflection, and discernment, and here this present volume from Maynooth seeks to make a small contribution.

The Pope's book uses the SEE-JUDGE-ACT process, familiar to many pastoral practitioners, based on the method proposed by Joseph Cardijn for the Young Christian Worker movement.[2] Pastoral and theological refection can benefit from these three stages. First, we contemplate the reality of our world, in this case, the pandemic. Second, we discern by uncovering what comes from God and promotes human dignity, as against what undermines it. And third, we propose suitable plans for action, based on that discernment.

Already in May 2020, Archbishop Eamon Martin appealed to Irish theologians and philosophers: 'I hope that philosophers, sociologists and media commentators of Ireland might begin to reflect on and critique how key societal relationships and partnerships have been impacted – for better or worse – by the pandemic. I encourage our theologians to consider what this crisis is saying to us about Church, about our identity and mission, about our relationship with the State, and about how prayer and faith can help sustain believers in a time of anxiety and crisis'.[3] In response, this volume provides reflections by members and associates of the theology and philosophy faculties of St Patrick's College, Maynooth.

The chapters are addressed to anyone seeking understanding,

---

2   See the Young Christian Worker website: ycw.ie/resources/see-judge-act-resources-2.
3   Archbishop Eamon Martin, *Homily for Ascension Sunday / World Communications Day*, 25 May 2020.

whatever their level of faith. The book seeks to assist those in parish ministry and interested laypersons, especially in the Irish context. Besides being valuable for personal reading, the volume is also intended as a resource for parish councils or small parish groups, because each chapter concludes with questions for reflection and discussion. This book seeks to offer the beginnings of a process of theological reflection that will doubtless take years to complete.

To be sure, this is not the only volume of theological reflections on the pandemic.[4] But the impact of the pandemic is so multifaceted that there is room to consider it from a variety of viewpoints. Accordingly, this volume offers a variety of reflections from the perspectives of philosophy, ethics, scripture, liturgy, pastoral theology, catechetics, history and canon law.

To set the scene, the volume begins with the insightful interview on COVID-19, given by Pope Francis to Austen Ivereigh, and published in *The Tablet* (8 April 2020). Thereafter, as in the Pope's 2020 book, *Let Us Dream*, the broad shape of this volume follows the SEE-JUDGE-ACT method. First, we look at the reality of the pandemic in church and society. Second, we discern what has been damaging and what has been life-giving during this difficult time. Third, we consider what we have learnt during the pandemic, leading to future action in response to the related social and religious changes.

The first stage of this volume is to see—to look at the pastoral, social, and religious realities of the pandemic. Reflecting on the experience of a particular church community in south Dublin, Anne Codd and Michael Hurley describe a parish journey through the current pandemic. Next, within pastoral reflections on the COVID-19 crisis, Aoife McGrath explores St Paul's image of the body of Christ

---

4   Pope Francis, *Life After the Pandemic* (Vatican City: Libreria Editrice Vaticana, 2020); Walter Brueggemann, *Virus as a Summons to Faith. Biblical Reflections in a Time of Loss, Grief and Uncertainty* (Eugene OR: Cascade Books, 2020); N. T. Wright, *God and the Pandemic: A Christian Reflection on the Coronavirus and Its Aftermath* (London: SPCK, 2020); Stephen Bullivant, *Catholicism in the Time of Coronavirus* (Park Ridge, IL: Word on Fire, 2020); Walter Kasper and George Augustin, eds., *Dios en la Pandemia* (Maliaño, Cantabria: Sal Terrae, 2020); Michael Heinlein and Harrison Ayre, *Finding Christ in the Crisis: What the Pandemic Can Teach Us* (Huntington, IN: Our Sunday Visitor, 2020).

and questions the temptation to simply put our Christian community living 'on hold' until the pandemic has passed. Michael Shortall considers the experience of grief at a time when public mourning is restricted, drawing both on published studies and on personal experience. Nóirin Lynch then offers a reality check, noting how COVID-19 has often reduced visible parish life to the priest's activity of live-streaming Mass. Finally, Salvador Ryan explores historical perspectives on the pandemic, asking whether the cessation of public Masses over several months because of COVID-19 might lead to the 'final rupture' in Irish religious practice.

The second stage concerns judging or discerning the meaning of the recent experiences. Here the chapters draw on the rich Christian heritage of scriptural, theological and philosophical reflection, composed during the many crises faced by people of faith through the generations. Two chapters explore scriptural resonances in the present crisis. In a chapter entitled, 'Singing the Lord's Song in a Strange Land,' Jessie Rogers considers the Jewish experience of lament in Psalms 77 and 137, while Jeremy Corley then explores how the Babylonian exile and the Jewish Sabbath may serve as helpful scriptural models for a time of pandemic. Facing the sharp question, 'Where is God in COVID-19?' Noel O'Sullivan engages with the difficult topic of theodicy, outlining the development of thinking about the problem of evil over the centuries. Two further chapters consider philosophical perspectives on COVID-19. Gaven Kerr reflects on God and the problem of suffering, drawing on the biblical story of Abraham and the works of Thomas Aquinas. Under the title, 'Retrieving Passion in the Pandemic: An Existential Response,' Thomas Casey creatively imagines how the great nineteenth-century philosopher Søren Kierkegaard might have reacted to the present crisis.

The third stage considers future action in response to the social and religious changes, in light of what we have learnt during the pandemic. Under the title, 'Do Not Be Afraid to Give Your Time to Christ,' Neil Xavier O'Donoghue explores the question of Sunday observance during a time of pandemic, seeking to open up the topic much wider than simply the Sunday Mass obligation. Thereafter, John-Paul Sheridan discusses some of the challenges of sacramental preparation online, noting the importance of children's experiences of God, especially in the domestic church. Pádraig Corkery then considers how, in an era of COVID-19, we may put into practice five challenging principles of Catholic Social Teaching: the common good, the universal destination of the world's goods, solidarity, subsidiarity and participation. Michael Mullaney explores sacramental and non-sacramental ways of encountering God's mercy in the extraordinary times of the pandemic, noting that the Church could allow general absolution in such circumstances. Kevin O'Gorman reflects on the significance, during a pandemic, of the prayer resource found in the Embolism of the Mass: 'Deliver us, Lord, we pray, from every evil.' Finally, Philip John Paul Gonzales seeks to develop a Christian metaphysics for the present era of COVID-19, proposing that a suitable response can be found in what he calls the 'foolishness of the daily'.

Three recurring themes run through this volume. The first theme concerns parish life during times of lockdown. While the provision of livestreamed Masses has served an important role, it is inadequate to think that parish life can be reduced to online liturgies, and there is a need to find creative means of involving many parishioners in the liturgical and pastoral life of each community. The second theme is the particular need to find ways to allow people to express their grief, especially at a time when public mourning is restricted. The third theme concerns the best human response to the pandemic, combining prayer, action for justice and continuing hopefully with our daily lives.

Overall, these chapters are intended to stimulate reflection and discussion, so that we can support one another during these difficult times and prepare to build a stronger future. No doubt each reader will be able to reflect on what they have taken from their reading of the various essays. We hope that ongoing reflection on the book's contents will lead to further understanding.

At this point, the editors would like to express thanks to many people who have helped the volume see the light of day. First of all, thanks are due to the President of Maynooth College, Rev. Prof Dr Michael Mullaney, for supporting this book project, and to the college's Scholastic Trust for generous financial assistance, which reduced the cover price of the book. Second, we are grateful to Austen Ivereigh and *The Tablet* for granting permission for the April 2020 interview with Pope Francis to be included in this volume. Third, thanks are due to the staff at Messenger Publications, especially Cecilia West (publisher), Donal Neary SJ (editor) and Paula Nolan (art director), for their professionalism and patience. Finally, as editors of the volume, we express our gratitude to all the contributors, who gave time to writing chapters.

We hope this volume will be helpful to lay Catholics, especially members of Parish Pastoral Councils, adult faith formation groups and parish discussion forums, as well as Catholic teachers and catechists; that it will benefit clergy and religious, especially preachers and retreat givers; and, finally, that it will assist anyone searching for spirituality during these difficult times.

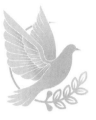

The Tablet Interview with Pope Francis on COVID-19, April 2020

Austen Ivereigh

*I*n an exclusive interview recorded for *The Tablet* (11 April 2020) – his first for a UK publication – Pope Francis told Austen Ivereigh that this extraordinary Lent and Eastertide [2020] could be a moment of creativity and conversion for the Church, for the world, and for the whole of creation.

Towards the end of March [2020], I suggested to Pope Francis that this might be a good moment to address the English-speaking world: the pandemic that had so affected Italy and Spain was now reaching the United Kingdom, the United States and Australia. Without promising anything, he asked me to send some questions. I picked six themes, each one with a series of questions he could answer or not as he saw fit. A week later, I received a communication that he had recorded some reflections in response to the questions. The interview was conducted in Spanish; the translation is my own.

The first question was about how he was experiencing the pandemic and lockdown, both in the Santa Marta residence and the Vatican administration ('the curia') more widely, both practically and spiritually.

POPE FRANCIS: The Curia is trying to carry on its work, and to live normally, organising in shifts so that not everyone is present at the same time. It's been well thought out. We are sticking to the measures ordered by the health authorities. Here in the Santa Marta residence we now have two shifts for meals, which helps a lot to alleviate the impact. Everyone works in his office or from his room, using technology. Everyone is working; there are no idlers here.

How am I living this spiritually? I'm praying more, because I feel I should. And I think of people. That's what concerns me: people. Thinking of people anoints me; it does me good, it takes me out of my self-preoccupation. Of course, I have my areas of selfishness. On Tuesdays, my confessor comes and I take care of things there.

I'm thinking of my responsibilities now, and what will come afterwards. What will be my service as Bishop of Rome, as head of the Church, in the aftermath? That aftermath has already begun to be revealed as tragic and painful, which is why we must be thinking about it now. The Vatican's Dicastery for the Promotion of Integral Human Development has been working on this, and meeting with me.

My major concern – at least what comes through my prayer – is how to accompany and be closer to the people of God. Hence the livestreaming of the 7am Mass [I celebrate each morning] which many people follow and appreciate, as well as the addresses I've given, and the 27 March event in St Peter's Square. Hence, too, the step-up in activities of the office of papal charities, attending to the sick and hungry.

I'm living this as a time of great uncertainty. It's a time for inventing, for creativity.

In my second question, I referred to a nineteenth-century novel very dear to Pope Francis, which he has mentioned recently: Alessandro Manzoni's *I Promessi Sposi* (*The Betrothed*). The novel's drama centres on the Milan plague of 1630. There are various priestly characters:

the cowardly curé Don Abbondio, the holy cardinal archbishop Borromeo, and the Capuchin friars who serve the lazzaretto, a kind of field hospital where the infected are rigorously separated from the healthy. In the light of the novel, how did Pope Francis see the mission of the Church in the context of COVID-19?

POPE FRANCIS: Cardinal Federigo [Borromeo] really is a hero of the Milan plague. Yet in one of the chapters he goes to greet a village but with the window of his carriage closed to protect himself. This did not go down well with the people. The people of God need their pastor to be close to them, not to over-protect himself. The people of God need their pastors to be self-sacrificing, like the Capuchins, who stayed close.

The creativity of the Christian needs to show forth in opening up new horizons, opening windows, opening transcendence towards God and towards people, and in creating new ways of being at home. It's not easy to be confined to your house. What comes to my mind is a verse from the *Aeneid* in the midst of defeat: the counsel is not to give up, but save yourself for better times, for in those times remembering what has happened will help us. Take care of yourselves for a future that will come. And remembering in that future what has happened will do you good.

Take care of the *now*, for the sake of tomorrow. Always creatively, with a simple creativity, capable of inventing something new each day. Inside the home that's not hard to discover, but don't run away, don't take refuge in escapism, which in this time is of no use to you.

My third question was about government policies in response to the crisis. While the quarantining of the population is a sign that some governments are willing to sacrifice economic wellbeing for the sake of vulnerable people, I suggested it was also exposing levels of exclusion that have been considered normal and acceptable before now.

POPE FRANCIS: It's true, a number of governments have taken exemplary measures to defend the population on the basis of clear priorities. But we're realising that all our thinking, like it or not, has been shaped around the economy. In the world of finance, it has seemed normal to sacrifice [people], to practise a politics of the throwaway culture, from the beginning to the end of life. I'm thinking, for example, of pre-natal selection. It's very unusual these days to meet Down's Syndrome people on the street; when the tomograph [scan] detects them, they are binned. It's a culture of euthanasia, either legal or covert, in which the elderly are given medication but only up to a point.

What comes to mind is Pope Paul VI's encyclical *Humanae Vitae*. The great controversy at the time was over the [contraceptive] pill, but what people didn't realise was the prophetic force of the encyclical, which foresaw the neo-Malthusianism which was then just getting underway across the world. Paul VI sounded the alarm over that wave of neo-Malthusianism. We see it in the way people are selected according to their utility or productivity: the throwaway culture.

Right now, the homeless continue to be homeless. A photo appeared the other day of a parking lot in Las Vegas where they had been put in quarantine. And the hotels were empty. But the homeless cannot go to a hotel. That is the throwaway culture in practice.

I was curious to know if the Pope saw the crisis and the economic devastation it is wreaking as a chance for an ecological conversion, for reassessing priorities and lifestyles. I asked him concretely whether it was possible that we might see in the future an economy that – to use his words – was more 'human' and less 'liquid'.

POPE FRANCIS: There is an expression in Spanish: 'God always forgives, we forgive sometimes, but nature never forgives.' We did not respond to the partial catastrophes. Who now speaks of the fires in Australia, or remembers that 18 months ago a boat could cross the North Pole because the glaciers had all melted? Who speaks now of the floods? I don't know if these are the revenge of nature, but they are certainly nature's responses.

We have a selective memory. I want to dwell on this point. I was amazed at the seventieth anniversary commemoration of the Normandy landings, which was attended by people at the highest levels of culture and politics. It was one big celebration. It's true that it marked the beginning of the end of dictatorship, but no one seemed to recall the 10,000 boys who remained on that beach.

When I went to Redipuglia for the centenary of the First World War I saw a lovely monument and names on a stone, but that was it. I cried, thinking of Benedict XV's phrase *inutile strage* ('senseless massacre'), and the same happened to me at Anzio on All Souls' Day, thinking of all the North American soldiers buried there, each of whom had a family, and how any of them might have been me.

At this time in Europe when we are beginning to hear populist speeches and witness political decisions of this selective kind, it's all too easy to remember Hitler's speeches in 1933, which were not so different from some of the speeches of a few European politicians now.

What comes to mind is another verse of Virgil's: *[Forsan et haec olim] meminisse iuvabit* ['Perhaps one day it will be good to remember these things too']. We need to recover our memory because memory will come to our aid. This is not humanity's first plague; the others have become mere anecdotes. We need to remember our roots, our tradition which is packed full of memories. In the *Spiritual Exercises* of St Ignatius, the First Week, as well as the 'Contemplation to Attain Love' in the Fourth Week, are completely taken up with remembering. It's a conversion through remembrance.

This crisis is affecting us all, rich and poor alike, and putting a spotlight on hypocrisy. I am worried by the hypocrisy of certain political personalities who speak of facing up to the crisis, of the problem of hunger in the world, but who in the meantime manufacture weapons. This is a time to be converted from this kind of functional hypocrisy. It's a time for integrity. Either we are coherent with our beliefs or we lose everything.

You ask me about conversion. Every crisis contains both danger and opportunity: the opportunity to move out from the danger. Today I believe we have to slow down our rate of production and consumption (*Laudato Si'*, 191) and to learn to understand and contemplate the natural world. We need to reconnect with our real surroundings. This is the opportunity for conversion.

Yes, I see early signs of an economy that is less liquid, more human. But let us not lose our memory once all this is passed, let us not file it away and go back to where we were. This is the time to take the decisive step, to move from using and misusing nature to contemplating it. We have lost the contemplative dimension; we have to get it back at this time.

And speaking of contemplation, I'd like to dwell on one point. This is the moment to see the poor. Jesus says we will have the poor with us always, and it's true. They are a reality we cannot deny. But the poor are hidden, because poverty is bashful. In Rome recently, in the midst of the quarantine, a policeman said to a man: 'You can't be on the street, go home.' The response was: 'I have no home. I live in the street.' To discover such a large number of people who are on the margins … And we don't see them, because poverty is bashful. They are there but we don't see them: they have become part of the landscape; they are things.

St Teresa of Calcutta saw them and had the courage to embark on a journey of conversion. To 'see' the poor means to restore their humanity. They are not things, not garbage; they are people. We can't settle for a welfare policy such as we have for rescued animals. We often treat the poor like rescued animals. We can't settle for a partial welfare policy.

I'm going to dare to offer some advice. This is the time to go to the underground. I'm thinking of Dostoyevsky's short novel, *Notes from the Underground*. The employees of that prison hospital had become so inured they treated their poor prisoners like things. And seeing the way they treated one who had just died, the one on the bed alongside tells them: 'Enough! He too had a mother!' We need to tell ourselves this often: that poor person had a mother who raised him lovingly.

Later in life we don't know what happened. But it helps to think of that love he once received through his mother's hope.

We disempower the poor. We don't give them the right to dream of their mothers. They don't know what affection is; many live on drugs. And to see them can help us to discover the piety, the pietas, which points towards God and towards our neighbour.

Go down into the underground, and pass from the hyper-virtual, fleshless world to the suffering flesh of the poor. This is the conversion we have to undergo. And if we don't start there, there will be no conversion.

I'm thinking at this time of the saints who live next door. They are heroes: doctors, volunteers, religious sisters, priests, shop workers – all performing their duty so that society can continue functioning. How many doctors and nurses have died! How many religious sisters have died! All serving ... What comes to my mind is something said by the tailor, in my view one of the characters with greatest integrity in *The Betrothed*. He says: 'The Lord does not leave his miracles half-finished.' If we become aware of this miracle of the next-door saints, if we can follow their tracks, the miracle will end well, for the good of all. God doesn't leave things halfway. We are the ones who do that.

What we are living now is a place of *metanoia* (conversion), and we have the chance to begin. So let's not let it slip from us, and let's move ahead.

My fifth question centred on the effects on the Church of the crisis, and the need to rethink our ways of operating. Does he see emerging from this a Church that is more missionary, more creative, less attached to institutions? Are we seeing a new kind of 'home Church'?

POPE FRANCIS: Less attached to institutions? I'd say less attached to certain ways of thinking. Because the Church is institution. The temptation is to dream of a de-institutionalised Church, a gnostic Church without institutions, or one that is subject to fixed institutions, which would be a Pelagian Church. The one who makes the Church is the Holy Spirit, who is neither gnostic nor Pelagian. It is the Holy Spirit who institutionalises the Church, in an alternative, complementary way, because the Holy Spirit provokes disorder through the charisms, but then out of that disorder creates harmony. A Church that is free is not an anarchic Church, because freedom is God's gift. An institutional Church means a Church institutionalised by the Holy Spirit.

A tension between disorder and harmony: this is the Church that must come out of the crisis. We have to learn to live in a Church that exists in the tension between harmony and disorder provoked by the Holy Spirit. If you ask me which book of theology can best help you understand this, it would be the Acts of the Apostles. There you will see how the Holy Spirit de-institutionalises what is no longer of use, and institutionalises the future of the Church. That is the Church that needs to come out of the crisis.

About a week ago an Italian bishop, somewhat flustered, called me. He had been going around the hospitals wanting to give absolution to those inside the wards from the hallway of the hospital. But he had spoken to canon lawyers who had told him he couldn't, that absolution could only be given in direct contact. 'What do you think, Father?' he had asked me. I told him: 'Bishop, fulfil your priestly duty.' And the bishop said *Grazie, ho capito* ('Thank you, I understand'). I found out later that he was giving absolution all around the place.

This is the freedom of the Spirit in the midst of a crisis, not a Church closed off in institutions. That doesn't mean that canon law is not important: it is, it helps, and please let's make good use of it, it is for our good. But the final canon says that the whole of canon law is for the salvation of souls, and that's what opens the door for us to go out in times of difficulty to bring the consolation of God.

You ask me about a 'home Church'. We have to respond to our confinement with all our creativity. We can either get depressed and alienated – through media that can take us out of our reality – or we can get creative. At home we need an apostolic creativity, a creativity shorn of so many useless things, but with a yearning to express our faith in community, as the people of God. So: to be in lockdown, but yearning, with that memory that yearns and begets hope – this is what will help us escape our confinement.

Finally, I asked Pope Francis how we are being called to live this extraordinary Lent and Eastertide [2020]. I asked him if he had a particular message for the elderly who were self-isolating, for confined young people and for those facing poverty as result of the crisis.

POPE FRANCIS: You speak of the isolated elderly: solitude and distance. How many elderly there are whose children do not go and visit them in normal times! I remember in Buenos Aires when I visited old people's homes, I would ask them: And how's your family? *Fine, fine!* Do they come? *Yes, always!* Then the nurse would take me aside and say the children hadn't been to see them in six months. Solitude and abandonment … distance.

Yet the elderly continue to be our roots. And they must speak to the young. This tension between young and old must always be resolved in the encounter with each other. Because the young person is bud and foliage, but without roots they cannot bear fruit. The elderly are the roots. I would say to them, today: I know you feel death is close, and you are afraid, but look elsewhere, remember your children, and do not stop dreaming. This is what God asks of you: to dream (Joel 3:1 [2:28]).

What would I say to the young people? Have the courage to look ahead, and to be prophetic. May the dreams of the old correspond to your prophecies – also Joel 3:1 [2:28].

Those who have been impoverished by the crisis are today's deprived, who are added to the numbers of deprived of all times, men and women whose status is 'deprived'. They have lost everything, or they are going to lose everything. What meaning does deprivation have for me, in the light of the Gospel? It means to enter into the world of the deprived, to understand that he who had, no longer has. What I ask of people is that they take the elderly and the young under their wing, that they take history under the wing, take the deprived under their wing.

What comes now to mind is another verse of Virgil's, at the end of Book 2 of the *Aeneid*, when Aeneas, following defeat in Troy, has lost everything. Two paths lie before him: to remain there to weep and end his life, or to follow what was in his heart, to go up to the mountain and leave the war behind. It's a beautiful verse. *Cessi, et sublato montem genitore petivi* ('I gave way to fate and, bearing my father on my shoulders, made for the mountain'). This is what we all have to do now, today: to take with us the roots of our traditions and make for the mountain.

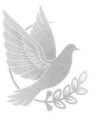

Becoming Church:
A Parish Journey into, through, and beyond the Pandemic

Anne Codd, PBVM and Michael Hurley

In December 2019 the parish newsletters of St Martin de Porres, Tallaght and Bohernabreena, neighbouring parishes in the south of the Archdiocese of Dublin, both of which are currently being served by the same parish team, carried the following:

> I have been part of the group gathering regularly over the last three months, exploring how our faith inspires us to reach out to each other and to our wider society, in a rapidly-changing context and culture. It has been a refreshing space, with time for chat and time for input on the mystery of our faith and the call to be Church today. ... Connection and sharing with each other are keys to building a faith community that sees the Spirit in action and inspires us to reach out, and we hope to encourage our communities to step out and reach out in love, celebrating the positive elements of our community as well as moving forward to meet future challenges.

Who could have imagined then what immediate and immense challenges, in the form of a global pandemic, we would be facing so soon afterwards? It is difficult to assess, as yet, the impact the pandemic will have in the longer term on faith, on religious practice and on Church life in general. Several surveys have been set in motion.[1] Processing the data, reflecting on the findings, and observing change as it unfolds will be ongoing.

Deprived of opportunities to express our belonging in communities of faith, questions arose. Joining in the communal prayer-life through liturgy and devotional practices was not an option. Deprived of ways to give witness to, as well as nourish, personal faith, what then could be said of one's core belief? And, very importantly, what does the Christian message, the Christian world-view, make of a pandemic?

Pastoral leaders are challenged to use every available means and opportunity to emphasise that the closure of church buildings does not mean the Church no longer exists. How aware are we of the mystery that, everywhere and at all times, for people of faith, it is 'in [God] that we live and move and have our being' (Acts 17:28)? What responsibility does human action have for the unfolding of God's creation – in this case into crisis?[2] How do we relate, in our present situation, to Christ as the 'first-born of all creation' (Col 1:15)? What is the difference between attending Mass streamed onto a home-screen and sharing in the Eucharistic celebration in-person as a community? What is the relationship between sacramental practice and the Christian belief that 'as long as you did it to the least of my [brothers or sisters] you did it to me' (Mt 25:40)? Can we not interpret family and neighbourly concern, as well as the selfless professionalism of front-line workers and services as – in truth – manifestations of divine graciousness?

In our own case, at a meeting of the core group of 'Co-responsi-

1   For example, under the Adult Religious Education and Faith Development Research Project, Mater Dei Centre for Catholic Education (MDCCE) at Dublin City University.
2   See Sean McDonagh, Columban eco-theologian, on human responsibility in this regard. www.columbans.ie/wp-content/uploads/2020/05/Worldwide-June-July-2020-PP12-13.pdf.

bility in Mission' in early September 2020, what emerged was that the public liturgies were being well managed, the voluntary supports were being sustained and, in some cases, cohorts were being augmented. Requests for help were also getting responses from 'newer' parishioners of non-Irish nationality.

It was clearly important to some parishioners to return to the communal celebration of Eucharist when restrictions were eased. At the same time, it was also acknowledged that the heart of liturgical celebration can be difficult to capture when so much attention has to be given to keeping at safe distances from one another and following rigorous directions.

Several pastoral initiatives were taken in the context of lockdown and restricted re-opening. Children receiving First Holy Communion, for example, received on the day a remembrance and a surprise 'package' on behalf of the community. Quietly, and in an almost unnoticed manner, community leadership (co-responsibility in mission) was taken and acted on. The celebrations of Confirmation, also under restrictions, were similarly carefully prepared for with willing cooperation of parents and teachers. The basics of stewarding and sanitising were part of the action. Reflection on the experience suggests that the sacramental celebrations were 'real and personal' – perhaps more so for the absence of some of the non-essential peripherals such as elaborate dressing up and the scale of gifts expected and received, which have been gaining undue importance for a long time now. It is as if some new seeds planted have been germinating in the dark of lockdown, and may yet produce fresh fruit of authentically faithful living.

The 'season of creation' (the weeks leading up to the Feast of St Francis on 4 October 2020) generated interest among some parishioners and connections were made through the media, with offers of time and prayer to be shared, even while physically remote from one another.

Limitations on meeting and movement and the need to 'wait and see' can be wearisome, and it is a challenge to sustain memory and hope. In this regard, the importance of resources for nurturing the life of the Spirit in faith and prayer and Christian living become ever more evident.

There has been an expressed need for the wholesome experience of being together again in person. On reflection, perhaps this desire for community is a very immediate and palpable proof of who we are as Church and what are some important values that we must preserve and nourish. It may also be a pointer to the key pastoral strategies that are being called for in our time – outreach and opportunity for human connection in safe and sustainable environments.

The journey to where we are now
The community at St Martin's was constituted a parish in 1985, having previously been part of the Dominican priory parish. In 2016 they celebrated the 40th anniversary of the official opening of their church. Bohernabreena parish comprises two communities; one is centred on the church of St Anne (the 'church on the hill'), which celebrated its sesquicentenary (150 years from foundation) in 2018, and the other on Holy Rosary Church, Ballycragh, which celebrated its 10th anniversary in 2019. These landmark dates are important indicators of the demographics of each community. The combined population of these church-area communities is some 20,000 people.

Among other developments in these communities there is one to which we wish to make special reference: with a recent reduction in the number of priests in the two parishes, one week-day morning Mass in each of the three churches has been replaced by a Service of the Word. Identifying leaders for these services has been greatly facilitated by having parishioners who participate in 'Cell Groups'.[3] While it is not easy to grow the practice of Services of the Word, we are convinced that they are essential to the life of local faith communities of the future.

---

3   At a time when many people are uncertain as to what they believe and unsure about how to share faith with others, cell communities offer a new beginning and a way forward for parishes and parishioners. A 'parish cell' is a faith community of 4 to 12 people, which offers support and faith formation. There are seven such communities within our parishes. See Michael Hurley, *Inspiring Faith Communities – A Programme of Evangelisation* (Dublin: Messenger Publications, 2020), with accompanying booklet, *Living Words*.

In co-authoring this piece, our hope is to share significant elements of our experience and in particular our reflections on what we are learning as we journey with three faith communities. We refer, where possible, to sources which have supported our theological and theoretical frameworks and the resources which have guided our practice. As parish priest, Michael is leader of the team which serves the communities and Anne has facilitated various stages of the developing process in recent years.

From maintenance to another way of being Church
The Parish Pastoral Councils (PPCs) of each of the two parishes completed their terms in 2018. These PPCs had served their communities admirably, in light of the circumstances of their time. Ministries and events were enabled as the needs arose. It is, however, common knowledge that enabling vibrant, missionary parish life has posed multiple and escalating challenges in Ireland for several decades now.

The evolution of the kind of Church envisaged by Pope Francis in what has been described as his 'manifesto' of 2013, *Evangelii Gaudium* (EG), is a demanding yet, we would say, exciting, task which, in the main, still lies ahead. A fundamental and long-term approach is needed. After much reflection, the team agreed that, guided by the documents published by the Irish Episcopal Conference in 2007 and 2011 as a framework for developing parish pastoral councils,[4] a working group would be convened by invitation. Those who had volunteered or been nominated for new PPCs would be included and, before the group would begin its work, the parish communities as a whole would be notified of its existence and task, and membership would be opened should other parishioners wish to join. The final membership of fifteen, including the parish team, was representative of the three communities and of their demographic spread. The

4   Episcopal Commission for Pastoral Renewal and Adult Faith Development, *Parish Pastoral Councils, a Framework for Developing Diocesan Norms and Parish Guidelines* (Dublin: Veritas, 2007); Irish Catholic Bishops' Conference, *Living Communion, Vision and Practice for Parish Pastoral Councils in Ireland Today* (Dublin: Veritas, 2011).

members were asked to commit to a monthly meeting for a six-month period.

This was a group with capacity for its purpose. The wisdom in the bishops' framework documents is evident. A 'working group' has a fixed term and a stated aim. The members can be selected in light of these, and at the same time provide the parish priest and team colleagues with broad perspectives from the community.

Crafting a statement of purpose

The conversations which took place in the early stages of the group's life were highly indicative of the diverse understandings and the range of expectations which are abroad in our communities. In terms used by congregational studies such as the ARCS project,[5] the mix of normative, formal, espoused and operant theologies of Church and ministry were very much in evidence.

In these conversations the following statement of purpose emerged:

> This group of 15, parishioners from three church areas together with our parish team, is invited to explore together how our communities can live and share the good news of God for the time and place in which we live.

Generating a shared vision

A chairperson from among the members of the working group was agreed and appointed. In addition to chairing the meetings, and so signalling group ownership of the task, this chairperson sat periodically with the parish team as they reviewed progress. In this way, the collaborative nature of the task, as well as the responsible leadership of the team, were sustained.

The meetings of the working group began, consistently, with a scriptural reflection mostly from the readings of the Mass of the day, with freedom for all to participate and to pray. In this regard, we were

---

5   ARCS, Action Research: Church and Society. See Helen Cameron et al., *Talking about God in Practice* (London: SCM Press, 2010).

following the wisest of advice, including that framed in strong clear terms by Loughlan Sofield and Carroll Juliano, widely acclaimed authors and enablers in pastoral development. What they recall saying to a Pastoral Council was entirely applicable to this working group:

> We shared our belief that a Pastoral Council is primarily engaged in discerning the will of God for the parish community. With this task as background, we encouraged them to spend at least a quarter of their meeting in prayer, reflection, and study. How is it possible to discern God's will without spending time in prayer?[6]

The group conversations were exploratory and inclusive, at once grounded and visionary, and by the fourth session a comprehensive ideal was emerging. The expansion of the 'dream' beyond the customary few sentences of a (seriously mis-named) 'mission statement' allowed the misgivings as well as the desires of the diverse membership to be aired, while drawing the basic orientation of the group into a shared direction. It was a service of leadership and facilitation to establish and hold the conversations within the parameters of Christian mission. The statement is admittedly schematised in light of the description of the early community in Acts 2:42, 44–45:

> They devoted themselves to the apostles' teaching and to fellowship, to the breaking of bread and to prayer [...] All the believers were together and had everything in common. They sold property and possessions to give to anyone who had need.

The dream we have found among us for our church area communities is that of being (Catholic) faith communities which:

---

6   Loughlan Sofield, S.T., and Carroll Juliano, S.H.C.J., *Principled Ministry: A Guidebook for Catholic Church Leaders* (Notre Dame, IN: Ave Maria Press, 2011).

- create welcoming spaces; spaces in which to talk; spaces in which to be silent;
- are marked by freedom and love;
- are communities to which people can belong, whether they are of majority or minority status;
- facilitate conversations on what matters; on what causes anxiety or fear.

We desire to grow continually as faith communities which:
- know that the news of our God is good;
- generate ways to share the good news and to welcome testimonies;
- are able to express what it is they believe, and why it is good news;
- are open to share life with communities of other churches (and faiths).

We recognise our call to be faith communities which:
- celebrate liturgy in ways that nourish faith, community and life; have necessary training for all who serve in public ministries; develop new ways to provide what is needed e.g. funeral and bereavement ministries, prayer leadership;
- have good organisation, so that Sunday liturgy can be celebrated well (and without stress);
- celebrate who they are in meaningful ways, using imagination and evoking emotions;
- celebrate in a variety of ways that reflect diverse ages (including children) and the interests of all in the community;
- generate experiences through creative use of music, poetry, art.

In our social context we wish to be faith communities which:
- are relevantly useful in our wider communities; share in a social and ecological agenda; learn from social action groups;

- know how to listen to all interests, to be attentive to what is real for people;
- are willing to ask searching and hard questions;
- can dialogue with a wide range of people and the alternative accounts of what life is about.

The working group recognised itself in the founding biblical text from Acts chapter 2, and equally the biblical text came alive in the group's reflections on itself as a community called to be Church.

In the fifth session, the group reached a significant juncture, triggered by the obvious question: who will hold and lead the communities in bringing this vision to life? The realisation dawned that while a dream is essential, it does not constitute a plan. The range of skills and resources which would be helpful in service of the vision was clear. The hard facts of pastoral life remain: there are fewer priests for the routine services that are expected, as well as for the range of crisis response which is often called for, in the widening geographic spread of emerging pastoral areas. There are also increasing (and legitimate) demands for good governance and administration. The service of permanent deacons and lay pastoral workers is welcome, but they too are numerically few.

Article 102 of *Evangelii Gaudium* came providentially to mind. There Pope Francis clarifies the centrality of the great (lay) majority of Church members in its missionary life. Also, and most importantly, he offers an analysis of why the gifts and potential commitment of most lay people for building up their faith communities lie dormant.

> Lay people are, put simply, the vast majority of the people of God. The minority – ordained ministers – are at their service. There has been a growing awareness of the identity and mission of the laity in the Church. We can count on many lay persons, although still not nearly enough, who have a deeply-rooted sense of community and great fidelity to the tasks of charity, catechesis and the celebration

of the faith. At the same time, a clear awareness of this responsibility of the laity, grounded in their Baptism and Confirmation, does not appear in the same way in all places. In some cases, it is because lay persons have not been given the formation needed to take on important responsibilities. In others, it is because in their particular churches room has not been made for them to speak and to act, due to an excessive clericalism which keeps them away from decision-making. Even if many are now involved in the lay ministries, this involvement is not reflected in a greater penetration of Christian values in the social, political and economic sectors. It often remains tied to tasks within the Church, without a real commitment to applying the Gospel to the transformation of society. The formation of the laity and the evangelisation of professional and intellectual life represent a significant pastoral challenge.(EG, 102)

While we were not, by a long stretch, the first or only people to recognise the wisdom enunciated by the Pope in this text, what was remarkable was the relevance of his words to our situation, the desire we had uncovered and the struggle we were experiencing. In this way, the text was not only *read*, it was *received* whole-heartedly – a clear example of the catechetical principle of the pivotal importance of readiness.[7]

The programme

It was very important that the parish team could tap the wisdom of the working group in drafting a formation programme. The pitch and the frequency, the duration and the timing as well as the content (the lyrics) and the methodologies that would be accessible for interested parishioners were ascertained through dialogue. As it turned out, while the enrolment of 15 participants (including some of the

---

7   Irish Catholic Bishops' Conference, *Share the Good News, National Directory for Catechesis in Ireland* (Dublin, Veritas, 2010)

working group) from across the three church areas was roughly half of what we had hoped for, the consistent attendance and participation throughout the course bore out the suitability of the plan.

It is opportune to quote here a second reflection by a participant, which indicates the content of the programme and which was also published in the newsletters of the two parishes:

> Over the last four months a group of parishioners from the three church areas (St Martin de Porres, Holy Rosary and St Anne's) have been taking part in a programme aimed at helping our communities to respond in faith to the changing times in which we live … The focus of the programme has been on what it means to live as a baptised Catholic today, how can we better share our faith and build up our communities as places of welcome, where people will come to know the Good News of Jesus in a way that speaks to our times. Using the teaching of Pope Francis from his document *The Joy of the Gospel* we have explored the Scriptures and the idea of the Church as a living, worshiping community at the service of others. In the new year we will be considering practical ways in which we can share these ideas and bring them to life in our church areas. It has been a privilege to be on this journey, to get to know one another better and to be enriched by the faith of all the participants.

In a 'review and planning' meeting in January 2020, facilitated by Fr Paddy Sweeney, a priest of Dublin archdiocese, uppermost in the conversation was what might be described as a 'felt memory' – the experience of the programme remained alive, treasured and inviting. The bonds which had formed were easily renewed. The commonality of belief, of gratitude and of mission were simply expressed. One remarkable feature of the entire journey, which carried over into this session, was the absence of judgement. From the outset, the group responded to the invitation to explore the mystery of our faith, and to allow the challenge of sharing the good news with others to emerge with time. This was refreshing.

In hindsight, it is utterly remarkable that Fr Paddy invited the participants to envisage what they had experienced as a viral infection! The burning issue was and remains: how are we to proceed in our emerging, area-based groups so that the mystery which we have glimpsed can become openly 'operant' in our communities, as the guiding force and the central feature of our witness?

Emerging structures and strategies

On Friday, 13 March 2020 – a date to remember – the conveners of the three area-based groups met as such for the first time with the parish team, as the core group of 'Co-responsibility in Mission'. They recounted their area groups' conversations during the previous two months and aired ideas for action that were emerging. There were two aspects to this meeting that we consider significant: firstly, we saw here the foundation of a structure for real collaboration in leadership, involving the parish team members, working in role, and parishioners with organic links into their respective communities; and secondly we noted how the unique characteristics of each community were being honoured within a shared mission.

The locus of responsibilities and the authority to make decisions of varying degrees of significance were key issues raised in the conversation. We discussed the relationships of the localised groups with others involved in services and ministries, as well as with their area communities themselves. We gave thought to the commitment which the conveners were being invited to give, and to the frequency and focus of meetings between the conveners and the parish team.

There was a strong desire among the smaller groups to have the full group of 15 together again, and also to have some further enrichment and encouragement. However, during our meeting there was a real sense of foreboding that something very serious was going on in our world, and that no one could know, for sure, how life would unfold in the days and weeks ahead.

It is noteworthy that just a month before (14 February), writing to Spain's National Congress for the Laity, Pope Francis was encouraging them to see themselves and the whole Church as:

> [the] emerging People of God [which] lives in a concrete history, which no one has chosen, but which is given to them, like a blank page on which to write. It is called to leave behind its comforts and take a step toward the other, trying to give a reason for hope (cf. 1 Pt 3:15), not with pre-fabricated answers, but with incarnated and contextualised ones, in order to make understandable and accessible the Truth that, as Christians, moves us and makes us happy.[8]

And then, the pandemic

A 'blank page on which to write' indeed! Within a few days the country was in pandemic lockdown, and public meeting places including churches were to remain closed. Existing communication networks – newsletters by email, WhatsApp groups, websites, Facebook and other social media were widely valued, and where these were underdeveloped, the need for them was recognised as urgent. In each of the three church areas, the emerging co-responsibility in mission groups became an important life-line for Michael and the parish team.

Opening up when the lockdown eased

Anecdotal evidence suggests that parishioners around the country responded handsomely to the call for volunteers to make possible the safe re-entry of community members into their church buildings. In our three church areas this was certainly the case. 'Co-responsibility in mission' was becoming a visible reality in a very practical way. The

---

8   Linda Bordoni, 'Pope urges lay Christians to go forth and make the voice of the Gospel resound', *Vatican News*, 14 February 2020, www.vaticannews.va/en/pope/news/2020-02/pope-message-laity-conference-spain-bishops.html.

willingness of parishioners to enlist for the range of services that was needed – notably in relation to health and safety and to technology – was remarkable, and their commitment is ongoing. The ownership of this project which is in evidence, is worthy of reflection. Is it a case of a new match in the parish community between needs and resources? Is it possible that the 'lay involvement' which has been genuinely desired by many pastoral leaders for years was perceived by most laity to be beyond their range? In the work which we have documented here, our experience is, in fact, of parishioners taking a step along the way from being fed and led to a readiness to feed and lead.

Looking ahead

It was providential that we had journeyed so recently and deliberately as a group of pastors and parishioners in conversations centred on how to become faith communities that are truly communities of missionary disciples. It helped to give, at least those involved, a sense of direction even in the context of an uncertain future.[9]

Questions for Reflection and Discussion

1. How far do the experiences described in this article find a parallel in your own parish?
2. The section on 'Generating a Shared Vision' outlines many elements of the 'dream' for the parish. How can the pastoral leadership of a parish enable, in their own context, some growth in each of the main areas (all essential) represented in the dream, while doing so in a harmonious way?
3. How can we encourage 'co-responsibility in mission' within our parish?

---

9   This chapter was written in September 2020, when restrictions had been lifted to an extent which allowed a limited reopening of churches.

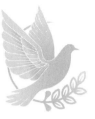

Suspended Animation?
Church in a Time of COVID-19

Aoife McGrath

We may try to understand the impact of the COVID-19 pandemic on our lives by using the lens of time. If we listen carefully to how people express their experience of the pandemic, embedded in these stories we can hear sentiments about time. Whether we are talking about a period of self-isolation, or the length of a local / national lockdown, or the duration of the pandemic itself, time is an important factor and discloses how we feel about and experience the pandemic: 'I can't see anyone or go anywhere for at least ten days, which means I have pretty much to stay in my bedroom to avoid the rest of my family for all that time'; 'I can't go "home-home" because I can't leave the county / go beyond 5km from my house for at least six weeks'; or, how revealing the phrase, 'when all this is over…'.

The pandemic itself has been called 'a fast-moving crisis' that requires an 'urgent', emergency-like response from everyone. Our government was challenged to 'move fast' and bypass typical procedures to effect changes in public policy, legislation, and expenditure. These changes have had an immediate impact on people's lives, on how we can spend our time and for how long, and what the long-term implications will be financially, emotionally, psychologically, and even physically.

For instance, we wonder what impact the increased time spent in lockdown will mean for victims of domestic violence, those with suicidal ideation, young adults who ought to be socialising and enjoying this time of their lives, elderly who feel abandoned by loved ones or cut off from friends because they have not seen them in so long, or those living alone with no human contact for extended – or more accurately, extending – periods of time. We also wonder what is the impact on the mobility and independence of our active-retired citizens who have lost their weekly social outings (such as dancing, bingo, or card-nights), or the elderly who are no longer permitted the agency to move about in public (to do their groceries, go to the post-office, meet their neighbours) or stay in control of their financial affairs, on a daily basis. The government's time-sensitive changes, in response to this fast-evolving pandemic, have impacted on our daily lives and our relationship with time itself.

As I write, we have entered a second national lockdown, expected to be of six weeks' duration – a period of regaining control over the spread of the virus so that we can break the chains of its transmission, and alleviate its negative impact on the Christmas period. It is a time of sacrifice and solitude now, in order that we might protect and guarantee the increase in intimacy of Christmas-time. This lockdown is widely expected to be a different experience from our first lockdown which took place in the spring–summer 2020. Since our clocks went back, the long dark evenings of winter-time and shorter daylight hours have given a different flavour to the lockdown experience this time around.

Practically since the pandemic began, people have been anticipating when it will be over – the global race for creating a vaccine and the time it will take to have it 'market-ready' are topics of many a conversation at the moment. Some speak of what life will be like 'post-COVID'; others are more focused on getting to post-lockdown, so that businesses can reopen and people can return to their jobs and social networks, and spend time with loved ones from whom we have been separated.

No less in faith communities, we hear people long for this COVID-time to be past. These communities too have had to make quick decisions, bypassing and transforming typical procedures, in response to the changing climate. This has meant rearranging and modifying the sacramental celebrations, facilitating near-private funeral ceremonies and burials, and broadcasting Masses online. These measures have been widely adopted, even if some people have objected to government restrictions on holding public religious services. Other measures are more difficult to quantify, as personnel and resources vary, and initiatives are not publicised or known beyond the respective community.

We may legitimately wonder, however, how many church activities have been suspended or curtailed to differing degrees across the country. The physical distancing required to minimise the risk of virus transmission and safeguard health services, school education and childcare, and protect vulnerable people and public health, complicates the interpersonal character of all Church activity. Suspending that activity beyond what is (sometimes unconsciously) deemed vital or essential, is the path of least resistance. That is not to say that there were no hurdles to surmount; in fact, there were plenty – technological dexterity, broadband access, caution when confronted with something new, suspicion of social media, fear of personal safety, or simply fatigue (and sometimes anger) in the face of yet another problem for faith practice.

Initially, given the short timeframe, quick decisions were made in the public health interest and various faith-based activities were inevitably limited. However, as the year has continued, and the pandemic lengthened, one has to wonder what continued Church decisions and remaining Church activities or practices tell us about what has been deemed essential from the Church's own perspective. The decisions of Church leaders, and their time-sensitive changes in response to government guidelines, are equally impacting the daily lives of Church members, our daily practice of faith, our relationship with one another, and thereby, ultimately, our relationship with God.

This is not to diminish the agency of Church members for the practice of their faith or the exercise of their discipleship. However, they legitimately look to Church leaders for encouragement, support, and spiritual nourishment, which the life, activity, and ministries of the Church are meant to sustain.

What has happened to those activities that were once deemed essential enough to warrant extensive time, energy, and resources, for the building of community and the nourishing of faith and discipleship? How many of them now 'survive' and what is the mode of this 'survival'? Do Pastoral Councils meet (even remotely), and if so, how often, and what now is their purpose or what are their tasks? Have children's liturgy or youth ministry practices ceased, or have they been transformed? What form of sacramental preparation, faith formation, care of the vulnerable, or social justice, if any, is taking place? Churches, like all people and organisations in this pandemic, have been impacted financially. As a consequence, in the Catholic Church certainly, the lay workforce has been significantly reduced. We may need to wait until the dust settles before it is truly known what Church activities have 'survived,' and indeed how many lay roles have been lost, whether paid or unpaid, part or full time, ministerial or administrative, at local, diocesan, and national levels.

A state of suspended animation?

The pace of life in general was forced to decelerate in our initial lockdown experience, and people took stock of their lives, reflecting on what they spend their time doing, and where they find meaning. Likewise, we must not neglect to reflect on our experience of Church, how we participate within it, and what part of it holds meaning for us. The danger of waiting for 'the COVID to be over,' is that Church bodies would quietly, inadvertently, or instinctively adopt a tactic of suspended animation where they slow down the life processes of our Church, to bide time and weather the COVID-storm. To be fair, the first lockdown brought about a sudden stop to virtually all activities in society – except for what was deemed essential for people's literal survival. That is not the case now, however. In public discourse, 'living with COVID' is the new mantra, and concerns for the developmental needs of children, and the needs of the elderly and the medically vulnerable, have been prioritised in the knowledge that life needs to continue. To what degree has 'living with COVID' infiltrated Church consciousness, I wonder? Certainly church buildings were adapted to comply with physical distancing measures, but what other steps have been taken to accept (if not embrace) a future with COVID-19? Have we even considered 'living with' a future of further novel coronaviruses or pandemics? I fear we run the risk of entering a state of hibernation now that reduces the functioning of the Church to a narrow definition of what is 'vital', which further leads us to think we can wait until 'the COVID' is over before the broader life and activity of the Church can recommence.

Neither survival nor mere maintenance can be an acceptable mode for a missionary Church in any era, even (and perhaps especially) in a pandemic era. In a time when people are contemplating the meaning of life in a whole new way, faith communities are called to give witness and communicate to others 'what has helped you to live and given you hope' (*Evangelii Gaudium*, 121), getting involved 'by word and deed in people's daily lives' (EG, 24).

St Paul was fond of using the image of the human body to communicate the relationship of Christ's disciples to one another and to Christ. If we take up that image, and consider the implications of what it might mean to focus the energy and life of the Church on what are considered 'vital' organs, this is what we might surmise: those parts of the body that are deprived of such life will eventually die. Think of how the body responds when exposed to extreme cold temperatures: in order to survive, the body protects its vital organs by slowing blood flow to the extremities so as to increase blood flow to the vital organs. As the blood is redirected away from the extremities, these parts of the body get colder, and fluid in the tissue can freeze and cause severe cell and tissue damage. The low blood flow also deprives the tissues of oxygen. If blood flow cannot be restored, these tissues will eventually die. This would be a dangerous path indeed if applied to the living body of the Church.

Contrast it with the following description from the first letter to Corinthians:

> The eye cannot say to the hand, 'I have no need of you,' nor again the head to the feet, 'I have no need of you'. On the contrary, the members of the body that seem to be weaker are indispensable, and those members of the body that we think less honourable we clothe with greater honour…. But God has so arranged the body, giving the greater honour to the inferior member, that there may be no dissension within the body, but the members may have the same care for one another. If one member suffers, all suffer together with it; if one member is honoured, all rejoice together with it. Now you are the body of Christ and individually members of it. (1 Cor 12:21–27)

Here Paul is trying to communicate something of the unity and diversity in the Church, which he refers to as the body of Christ. The passage shows how all parts of the body should be equally indispensable, or vital. The suffering of one part affects the whole. If anything, COVID-19 has provided ample confirmation that we are interdependent beings. This is no less true in the body of the Church; we each cannot live without one another.

The Decree on the Apostolate of the Laity from November 1965 springs to mind, where the Council Fathers unequivocally stated: 'no part of the structure of a living body is merely passive but has a share in the functions as well as life of the body: so, too, in the body of Christ, which is the Church, "the whole body … in keeping with the proper activity of each part, derives its increase from its own internal development" (Eph. 4:16)'[1]. To me, if our approach during COVID-

---

1   *Apostolicam Actuositatem* (18 November 1965), http://www.vatican.va/archive/hist_councils/ ii_vatican_council/documents/vat-ii_decree_19651118_apostolicam-actuositatem_en.html.

19 treats or relegates lay people to a merely passive role – making them bystanders or spectators in the life and activity of the Church – then there is something seriously amiss with our perception of what is vital within the living body that is the Church.

Even if we argued that such measures might be temporarily necessary, while waiting for COVID-19 to be over, waiting for Christians is not something undertaken in a state of suspended animation. For Christians are not averse to the experience of anticipation and waiting. We are an eschatological people after all, waiting in hopeful expectation and anticipation of the second coming of Christ. Indeed, during the approach to the season of Advent, we share in the preparation for Christ's first coming and renew our expectancy of his second coming. In the lead-up to Advent, we hear once again the 'parable of the ten bridesmaids' (8 November 2020), and the 'parable of the talents' (15 November 2020). These parables prompt us to ask the question – how should we, as Christians, spend a time of waiting and anticipation? The answer – stay awake, be alert and ready; do not bury the gifts you have been given in the ground, rather invest time and energy so that they will bear fruit. Waiting, for Christians, is therefore a time of activity and animation. It is a time when people are given and accept responsibility for their share in a mission that is as important in this moment, as it ever was.

A place and a part for everyone

If the image of the body does not hold sufficient meaning for understanding the Church, let me try another: the jigsaw puzzle. This analogy is limited in its own way, but it has been sitting with me, in my semi-isolation, since COVID-19 first appeared. During that time, I have completed three jigsaw puzzles – all sent to me as gifts in the post, all with 1,000 pieces, and all Harry-Potter-themed (in case you were curious). As a budding puzzle enthusiast, I have acquired a systematic approach for completing the task which rarely fails me. It is not rocket science: I simply start with the 'edge pieces' to complete the frame and, following the pattern, work my way towards the centre.

I find it remarkable how each piece is uniquely designed to fit its particular place in the puzzle, a perfect fit with its surrounding companions. If I were to place a piece in the incorrect position, first it would simply not fit – and would mean forcing a piece into a position where it just does not belong; and second, it could set the whole project astray for however long it would take me to realise my error and set the wrong to rights (neither of which happened, pride obliges me to tell you). If I were to damage or lose a piece, the puzzle would be ruined entirely (that's the perfectionist in me, but, I can assure you, this did not happen either, even if the fear was palpable). As I sat during lockdown, methodically building each jigsaw puzzle, time was of no concern to me: sure, where else did I have to be? When I sent pictures of my progress to some friends, they admired my patience. However, for someone who is enthusiastic about puzzle-making, I only felt a quiet and peaceful joy, and a certain amount of fulfilment in seeing the fruits of my labours.

It occurred to me how puzzle-making could be a useful analogy for building community within the Church. Each person is uniquely created to fulfil a particular task, sharing in the common purpose of the whole, beautifully contributing to and completing the grand design for which they were created. Meditative and engaged discernment is necessary to identify each person, recognise his / her gifts, and find his / her place within the whole. Lest this imply that those in ministerial leadership stand in the place of the puzzle-maker, independently prescribing the place of each, we must remember that we speak of the people of God and not objects. Therefore, the task of those in leadership is to accompany people in the exercise of communal discernment in finding the place (and part) God calls each to take up within the whole. Indeed, ministers 'initiate everyone – priests, religious and laity – into this "art of accompaniment"' (EG, 169), so that we accompany one another in this discernment and in fulfilling our particular vocation. If someone were lost, or ignored, or excluded, the community as a whole would suffer. Trying to complete the puzzle with fewer pieces, placing them where they are not meant to go, speaks to me of focusing on only a few within the community and trying to fit them together without reference to others. This likewise diminishes the whole and fails to serve the purpose for which it was created, and to which it is called.

Of course, one primary advantage I had in building my jigsaws was having prior knowledge of the overall pattern or design. With the box cover propped up in front of me, how could I fail to place each piece correctly, eventually? Those building community have no such luxury. We have a sense of God's plan and the end for which we are reaching, but we have no direct blueprint to indicate who should go where or do what. The Spirit is our guide and careful communal discernment all the more important.

But even if we do not have the exact pattern, that is not to say that we should give up on the task. As my mother rightly remarked, it helped that I was so familiar with the subject matter of the puzzles – I knew where to put the pieces without seeing the picture. This was a truth I could not deny; more often than not, I did not have to consult the box at all because I knew the characters: the colour of their hair, the clothes they wore, what they were likely to have in their hands, even the expression they were likely to have on their faces. In short, I knew where to place the puzzle pieces, because I knew their story and the story of which they formed a part. It brought home to me the need for familiarity in community building, the need to know the story of each person – and not just his / her need, but his / her gift, and where that gift might fit in the overall story.

That is all well and good, you might say, but we are in the midst of a pandemic, where time is short, and decisions must be made urgently. In response, I recall Pope Francis's assertion in his 2013 document on 'The Proclamation of the Gospel in Today's World': 'Here we see a first principle for progress in building a people: time is greater than space' (EG, 222). He continued:

> This principle ... helps us patiently to endure difficult and
> adverse situations... It invites us to accept the tension

between fullness and limitation, and to give a priority to time. ... Giving priority to time means being concerned about initiating processes rather than possessing spaces. Time governs spaces, illumines them and makes them links in a constantly expanding chain, with no possibility of return. What we need, then, is to give priority to actions which generate new processes in society and engage other persons and groups who can develop them to the point where they bear fruit in significant historical events. Without anxiety, but with clear convictions and tenacity. (EG, 223)

The principle of giving priority to time takes on new meaning during a worldwide pandemic emergency. It opposes the notion that we bide our time, and suspend animation, until the crisis is over. Rather, it challenges us to give priority to actions that generate new processes, and to engage others who can develop these processes and take up their part in the service of the ultimate purpose to which we are called. For the Church, 'building a people' is still this purpose – to offer our lives to others in mission, so that we may be 'gathered together as one' (*Lumen Gentium*, 13) – even in a time of COVID-19.

The urgency of the pandemic has directly had an impact on the progress of this mission in our contemporary world. It has played with our sense of time and space – state leaders have had limited time in which to consider, decide, and urge collective responsibility and action to change the patterns of virus transmission. For the rest of the population, often confined to our homes or within a limited radius, time has seemed endless while we wait for the periods of self-isolation, lockdown, or the pandemic to pass. Within the Church, leaders have quickly responded, adapting our physical church spaces, while adopting new technologies to transform the Church's presence in online spaces.

However, given the real risk that quick decisions may occasion a growing passivity among the lay faithful, we need to prioritise careful communal discernment that finds new ways to engage (rather than disengage) people, enabling them to take up their place and part in our shared mission. We should not be placing our energies in spaces where the focus is on a few to the detriment of the whole. Rather, we need to work patiently, even in a challenging COVID-landscape, to enable others to discover their place and active part in the life of discipleship, in the spaces where they find themselves. This will require careful listening to others, becoming familiar with their stories, and engaging deeply with the impact of COVID-19 on their lives. We do well to remember, however, that we are not merely discerning their need so that a few can offer the active response. Instead, in compassionate listening, we accompany and enable them to find their own path, and generously share the gifts they have received for the good of all.

Questions for Reflection and Discussion

1. How has 'COVID-time' been for you personally? What stories do you have to share from your COVID experience?
2. Are you aware of any quick decisions or changes to typical approaches within your faith community? If so, what do you think is the impact of these decisions and changes, in the short, medium, and long-term?
3. Is the notion of 'suspended animation' useful for characterising the life of your faith community during COVID-19? If so, what activities do you think have been suspended or curtailed? Have some lay roles been reduced or lost?
4. What is the most visible representation of parish life in your locality at present? Who is most involved in these activities and what is their role?
5. In what practical ways do you think your parish or pastoral area could transform its activity in order to 'live with COVID-19'

rather than simply 'biding time until it is over'?

6. What place do you hold, and what part do you animate, within your local faith community? Who do you think accompanies you in your involvement, and how do they accompany you?

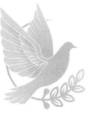

Grief Observed When Mourning Is Restricted

Michael Shortall

'No-one ever told me grief would feel so like fear.' So goes the opening line of *A Grief Observed* written by C.S. Lewis in 1961. He continued: 'I am not afraid, but the sensation is like being afraid.'[1] Nearly sixty years later, fear weaved itself more forcefully into the experience of grief and mourning. In March 2020, people in Ireland were afraid. The global pandemic of COVID-19 reached Europe. At first, we watched events unfold in Italy and Spain. Then quite suddenly, in the space of days, restrictions were announced. On 12 March, schools and colleges were shut, and large gatherings were advised to cancel, including public worship on Sundays. Within two weeks, almost all businesses and facilities were shut, non-essential travel banned, and the elderly and vulnerable told to cocoon. Yet the virus took hold. As hospitals and elderly-care homes quarantined, many people died without loved ones being present and their loved ones, in turn, experienced a restricted grief and mourning.

A few pages later, Lewis wrote:

> And grief still feels like fear. Perhaps, more strictly, like suspense. Or like waiting; just hanging about waiting for

---

1 C.S. Lewis, *A Grief Observed* (London: Faber & Faber, 1964), 1.

something to happen. It gives life a permanently provisional feeling. It doesn't seem worth starting anything. I can't settle down. I yawn, I fidget, I smoke too much. Up till this I always had too little time. Now there is nothing but time. Almost pure time, empty successiveness.[2]

As the months stretched into the summer and autumn, these lines seemed strangely apt. Even though restrictions eased somewhat, society hung in a kind of 'suspense' between two experiences of time. People regularly spoke of how the months slipped by quickly, even as the days passed slowly. It is reminiscent of Lewis's experience of mourning or grieving. After all, so much was lost – jobs, education, sport and new experiences. And more importantly, so many had died.

A Grief Observed has become a classic in the genre of memoirs concerning bereavement. It is a short series of reflections on the experience of bereavement after Lewis's wife, Joy Davidman, died of cancer. He had already gained popularity as the author of a series of fantasy novels – *The Chronicles of Narnia* – and as a Christian apologist. In this book he explores his emotional responses, the changes to his life and the questions it raised for his faith. Other autobiographies are equally compelling and moving: *In Memoriam* (1980) is a moving account by Henri Nouwen of the sudden illness and death of his mother from cancer[3]; *Lament for a Son* (1996) is written with searing honestly by Nicholas Wolterstorff on coming to terms with the loss of his 25-year-old son in a mountain climbing accident[4]; and *The Year of Magical Thinking* (2005) by Joan Didion is a masterful work about the death of her husband and the severe illness of her daughter.[5]

As the title of Lewis' book – *A Grief Observed* – makes clear, it tells one person's experience. The uniqueness of each experience is confirmed by other accounts. Yet, they powerfully resonate with readers, because grief and mourning are universal. It is possible to recognise

---

2   Lewis, *A Grief Observed*, 15.
3   Henri Nouwen, *In Memoriam* (Notre Dame, IN: Ave Maria Press, 1980).
4   Nicholas Wolterstorff, *Lament for a Son* (Grand Rapids, MI: Eerdmans, 1996).
5   Joan Didion, *The Year of Magical Thinking* (New York: Random House, 2005).

tendencies and processes through which people manage loss. The intent of this chapter is to chart the dynamic of grief and mourning, and to reflect on the impact of restrictions on its process.

Models of mourning and grieving

Let us begin by considering some distinctions between bereavement, grief and mourning. Bereavement, firstly, refers to the fact of loss itself. Grief implies the subjective response. It is the personal stress reaction to a real, perceived or anticipated loss. It may occur where there is any loss: such as a death, significant injury or loss of a relationship or property; or, less tangibly, the loss of purpose. While its intensity is individual, it is not inevitable. It is possible to be bereaved and not to grieve. Mourning, finally, has two meanings. It may refer to the process of grieving whereby a person adapts to loss. It may also refer to the social behaviours, norms and rituals by which grief is recognised and processed, such as wearing black, giving flowers and so on. These two aspects can be interrelated and so influence one another. As a result, if certain accepted social practices are not adhered to, the personal process of adaptation can be arrested. For example, if the body, grave or urn cannot be seen, the capacity to accept the reality of the death of a loved one can be impeded.

There have been a number of approaches to mapping the psychological processes or progression of grief.[6] As we have noted, because grief and mourning can be highly individual, it is difficult to tease out patterns. The manifestations of grief can be complex, with physical, emotional, cognitive, spiritual, behavioural and indeed cultural components. Contemporary models emphasise that it is a natural response and it can continue in different forms even after adaption to loss. Other approaches highlight the way in which grief can lead to a reconstruction of the self, relationships and spirituality. In other words, while a painful process, it also may be a catalyst for growth.

The most well-known model is that first proposed by Elizabeth

---

6   See Therese A. Rando, *How to Go on Living When Someone You Love Dies* (New York: Bantam Books, 1991).

Kübler-Ross in *On Death and Dying*.[7] While her model has entered into popular knowledge and culture, it is worth recalling. She suggested five stages identifiable in the dying and those grieving the dead. The first stage of significant loss is denial, in which the individual struggles to accept the reality of the situation. The fact of loss seems mistaken or false or unbelievable, allowing for another preferred reality to be created and clung to. However, with reality coming to bear, the person becomes frustrated, especially with others close to them. It overflows into the second stage of anger, questioning, blaming and a sense of injustice. The third stage moves to an attempt to negotiate a way through the fear or pain. In grieving death, it can manifest as pondering 'if only', with consequent feelings of guilt. During the fourth stage, recognition of mortality or finality hits home. The person can retreat into themselves, becoming sad and sullen. In the final stage, mortality of another – or indeed oneself – is accepted, leading to a more stable balance of emotions.

In spite of its popularity, further research over the past half-century has not corroborated this model. In particular, grief does not follow a linear pathway or timetable. While recognising the different types of manifestations of grief is important, a stages approach to mourning should not be over-stressed.[8] It can give the impression there is a single way to 'grieve rightly'. Today, accounts of this model always come with a disclaimer that the stages do not have to follow a specific order. A person can move back and forth between them, and indeed skip a stage. However, and more importantly, the most significant criticism of a stages approach is that it can give the impression that the individual is passive. There is now greater understanding that the participation or efforts of the individual are required. The griever needs to find a way, even it is only 'to muddle through', slowly building capacity to make sense of loss and reconnect with the deceased.

Instead of stages, William Worden in *Grief Counselling and Grief*

---

7 Elizabeth Kübler-Ross, *On Death and Dying* (New York: Macmillan, 1969).
8 Colin Murray Parkes suggested four stages: shock, angry pining, depression and despair, and detachment. See Colin Murray Parkes, *Bereavement: Studies of Grief in Adult Life*, 4th ed. (New York: Routledge, 1972, 2010).

Therapy (1991) describes four tasks in grieving.[9] The first task of the griever is to recognise the reality of loss, that is, come to accept the actuality of the event. Secondly, the griever needs to deal with the wide range of expressed and latent feelings that can arise in grief. Thirdly, the griever needs to endeavour to live in the world without the deceased by adjusting to new realities. The realities may be external such as new responsibilities and roles: for example, new parenting roles after the death of a spouse or a partner for someone with a young family. The realities may also be internal: for example, the spouse may experience new feelings of loneliness. Finally, the griever needs to find how to work through a way of relocating the deceased in one's life while moving on. This last task reaffirms that the relationship is not in fact over but reimagined and reappropriated. Social and ritual practices are vital in the undertaking of grief. They provide the expectations and norms for what is to be done when death impacts a griever. While for some they can feel oppressive, they can also transmit the wisdom and support of the community.

Worden's four tasks are recognisable in many traditional Irish funeral practices. A straightforward example of how the first task of recognising the reality of loss is supported and reinforced is the practice of 'viewing the body' in an open coffin at home. We can notice the second task at work in the socially acceptable spaces that occur in the relatively large gatherings for strong, overpowering, confused and indeed intimate feelings to be expressed publicly. A strong community context – and the friendships it fosters – is more likely to provide support beyond the funeral rites for the third task of navigating new roles in life. The final task of remaining connected with the deceased and the beliefs is evident in a range of practices, such as gatherings for anniversaries and the care of the grave.[10]

The individual is required to engage with these tasks if the normal process is not to stall into 'complicated grief'. It has been estimated

9   William Worden, *Grief Counselling and Grief Therapy* (London: Routledge, 1991).
10 For this in an Irish context see Salvador Ryan (ed.), *Death and the Irish: a Miscellany* (Dublin: Wordwell, 2016).

that about seven per cent of people develop 'complicated grief,' or intense and exaggerated responses to loss that effectively impair a person's capacity to function well.[11] It can be reinforced when there is no social acknowledgement or space for grief to be openly mourned. This restriction may be described as a 'disenfranchised grief': examples include where the loss is not recognised (e.g. a pet), the relationship is not acknowledged (a friend), the griever is not acknowledged (a child or person with a disability), the death causes shame (e.g. suicide), or if manifestations of grief are considered inappropriate (e.g. cultural differences).

In mid-March 2020 Ireland went into lockdown. Funerals and mourning practices were suddenly and substantially impacted. How would society manage grieving, when many of the customary social and ritual practices became unavailable so abruptly?

A personal experience
My father died during the lockdown. He didn't die of COVID-19; but his care and dying, and our mourning, were all shaped by it. Some rituals had to be abandoned; others, because of technology, took on new forms.

In life, Dad took seriously the responsibility of going to funerals. Of course, there was the social aspect, the obligatory raising of a glass in honour of someone. But it was also to use an old phrase, a corporal work of mercy: 'to pray for the dead'. This obligation can be especially strong in rural areas, like my home in northern Kilkenny. It is a community as much as a family that loses someone. But suddenly, the community couldn't do the same for him – well, certainly not in the same way. Only ten family members were permitted to be present at 'the viewing of the body' and the Requiem Mass. I can still see the big wooden doors of the church shutting behind us, allowing no-one else in. To say we felt robbed or cheated can imply that there is someone to blame. There isn't. From a public health perspective, the

---

11 See: M. Katherine Shear, 'Grief and mourning gone awry: pathway and course of complicated grief,' *Dialogues in Clinical Neuroscience* 14/2 (2012) 119–128.

restrictions were appropriate. Yet, we really felt the lack of a normal funeral. We were to some degree disenfranchised, to use the language of the literature. The peculiarly Irish rituals weren't available to us, to our neighbours and friends, and most of all to Dad.

Yet we adapted as best we could, and technology helped hugely. 'We had a small funeral. Half the world was there', my mother would say afterwards. It was striking how many people tuned in to the live stream on the parish website. It helped my sister especially, who lives abroad and couldn't make it home. She was even able to participate, as she led a decade of the family rosary on a smart phone, from three thousand miles away.

The community did what they could too. Some neighbours stood respectfully at a long distance in the graveyard under the sunshine for the burial. We returned to our home to find food left outside our door. The phone continually rang for days. So many condolences were shared on the rip.ie website. Sympathy cards kept coming. And then everything went quiet until the restrictions eased a little and the first people started to visit. But not many came. As the restrictions stretched on and on, neither my sister nor family from across Ireland could travel easily.

The death notices on local radio are very much part of rural life. Each one finished with a line saying in effect, 'a memorial will be held at a later date'. It reminded me of a litany. I don't think many grieving families realised how much later the memorial would be.

A Christian reflection

So how did society manage grieving? The answer is like grieving itself; it muddled through as best it could.

But there are concerns. The long-term imposition of the restrictions may alter the social practices that facilitate the process of grief. In particular, it may weaken communal customs and traditions, and lead to a privatisation of mourning, often experienced in other countries. This trend, facilitated by urbanisation, is already noticeable in the larger cities. The response to COVID-19 may hasten this disquieting development.

Catholic funeral and mourning practices are underpinned by a perspective on grief and, more fundamentally, an understanding of what it means to be human in relation to the divine. From this viewpoint, grief is not a private affair, a trauma to be solved, reducible to a therapeutic process. Rather it is a fully human experience. I would like to suggest four important elements to a Christian approach to the experience of loss. Taken together, they warn and argue against the continued privatisation of mourning.

First, loss is expressed as lamentation. The scriptures present many examples of loss being articulated through a full range of emotion. Lamentation demands that our emotions of sadness be expressed and articulated, even if it means complaint, blame and anger is to be directed at God. For example, nearly a third of the Psalms can be described as lamentations. 'You have put me into the depths of the Pit, in the regions dark and deep' (Ps 88:7). Or: 'Out of the depths I cry to you, O Lord. Lord, hear my voice! Let your ears be attentive to the voice of my supplications!' (Ps 130:1–2)[12]

Secondly, Christian belief attests that loss – as an element of suffering – is integral to life itself. The Paschal Mystery, that is, the death and resurrection of Jesus, puts loss and consequent grief at the very centre of the God's salvific action. Mourning and grief should not be denied or compartmentalised, not only because it is psychologically unhealthy, but because it is the place in which the crucified God can be revealed. Pope Francis in *Gaudete et Exsultate* (2018), written on the theme of holiness, turned to the theme of mourning in reflecting on the Beatitude, 'Blessed are those who mourn, for they will be comforted.' (Mt 5:4) He observes:

> The world has no desire to mourn; it would rather disregard painful situations, cover them up or hide them. Much energy is expended on fleeing from situations of suffering

---

12 The role of lamentation is further explored by other contributors to this collection.

in the belief that reality can be concealed. But the cross can never be absent. (GE, 75)

Thirdly, loss is a deeply social concern. While death is a profoundly unique individual experience, grief and mourning are necessarily relational. After all, someone is emotionally reacting to the loss of another. But as social beings, people require a network of relationships by which to navigate a new reality without someone. While the social practices regarding mourning are vital to a healthy society, in a Christian light it is also a matter of lived discipleship. To have concern for our neighbour is the practical expression of the concern of God. This is why Pope Francis could conclude the above passage in *Gaudete et Exsultate* so concisely: 'Knowing how to mourn with others: that is holiness' (GE, 76).

Fourthly and finally, loss is hope-filled. St Paul writes to the church in Thessalonica: 'But we do not want you to be uninformed, brothers and sisters, about those who have died, so that you may not grieve as others do who have no hope.' (1 Thess 4:13) Paul goes on to provide a vision of the final times when Christ will return and gather all to himself. He concludes 'Encourage each other with these words.' (1 Thess 4:18). Paul did not say, 'don't grieve at all'. Rather, the muddled, emotional pendulum of grief is placed in a new context. Indeed, the fact that death is not the end provides space for grief to be fully experienced. Without hope, grief can too easily become self-pity or despair, rather than the recognition and honour to a loved one that it is.

C.S. Lewis mentions the above line from St Paul in *A Grief Observed*. He reacts angrily to it when it is used as a 'consolation of religion,' in phrases like: 'family reunions on the further shore,' 'She is at peace now,' 'She is in God's hands now.'[13] Instead, he wants to name the reality of what he is going through. Later however he admits, 'I thought I could describe a state; make a map of sorrow.

---

13 Lewis, *A Grief Observed*, 13.

Sorrow, however, turns out to be not a state but a process. It needs not a map but a history'.[14]

At the beginning of this reflection, an analogy was made between grief and the experience of Irish society as it experienced the pandemic of COVID-19 and the subsequent restrictions. Lewis's conclusion then might also be apt. 'Roadmaps' entered our language in the government response when trying to leave lockdown. They were necessary in charting a way through a potentially horrific situation. Yet, attention to what people were actually going through is vital. When the guidelines pass away, the experience of the pandemic – including those who grieved lost ones – will require articulation. It is the personal history of what happened. Could the Church, in its calling to be an agent of healing in the world, be that place where people can speak, remember and ritualise how they 'muddled through'?

Questions for Reflection and Discussion

1. Did you have an experience of a funeral during the lockdown? What was it like for you?
2. How might the five stages of grief, outlined by Elizabeth Kübler-Ross, resonate with your own experience?
3. Can you identify other religious rituals or social practices that aid the four tasks of mourning listed by William Worden?
4. The Scriptures again and again show lamentation as a response to loss. Our emotions, including anger or upset, can be directed at God. Recalling a loss in your life, what did you say to God? What might you say now?
5. Grief and mourning are also a time in which God can work in our lives. Through that process we can come to new understandings or freedom or maturity. Can you name how this might have happened in your life?

---

14 Lewis, *A Grief Observed*, 28.

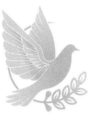

Keeping Fathers Busy: COVID, Clericalism and Parish Life

Nóirin Lynch

It feels surreal and even unfair to speak of parish life during the COVID-19 crisis, as in truth we are still writing from the middle of a pandemic, not from hindsight! How can one offer a fair perspective or a critique, when so many are doing all they can in truly challenging circumstances?

Perhaps the only gift a reflection like this might offer is a fresh perspective on how we can live well as Christians in this new reality: a perspective to help us avoid both the attraction of busyness and the despair of inaction. The old maps no longer work[1], and yet, like the three visitors from the east, we can find our way even if in a different way from what we expected (Mt 2:12).

Let me start by saying that yes, the Irish Church has visibly worked to develop parish pastoral development for decades. However, this crisis has revealed our priorities. Have we prioritised Mass over meetings, sacrament over family prayer, familiarity over creativity? Not all these things are bad, but have we moved from a focus on empowering faith communities into one of keeping our clergy busy? As Bishop Donal Murray prophetically remarked in 2005 at a Chrism Mass in Limerick:

---

1   'Old Maps No Longer Work', by Joyce Rupp, OSM, online: vimeo.com/315916263.

... (if) any of us were to imagine that the life of the parish or the diocese was meant to be the fruit simply of our (priests') gifts and our ideas and our (priests') way of doing things we would be settling for an impoverished, lifeless community.[2]

In this chapter I'd like to consider how this crisis has revealed an operative spirituality that is more privatised and clerical than we might like to believe. I know that the desire for inclusive, inspiring parish life exists. We deserve good leadership now to encourage us in necessary reflection and action as we plan. I also offer some questions / ideas for a way ahead.

Knowing who we are

If we are to speak of how we lead, we need to start with who we are. I begin with Eucharist for two reasons: because it is the heart of who we are, and because it is also where the primary effort of parish life seems to have focused in these past months.

Eucharist is at the heart of who we are – our inspiration and our sustenance.[3] In the lived experience of parish life, however, what we mean by that is not always clear: is the role of Eucharist to offer a comforting space for some lay people, or is it to develop a eucharistic culture that stretches beyond our personal needs into discipleship for the whole world?[4]

During this COVID-19 crisis, two different understandings of ourselves as a eucharistic people have been visible in Irish parish life, each with their own consequences.

The first understanding, often referenced in an academic setting or in pastoral development work, is that, gathered as Eucharist, we recognise ourselves as the Body of Christ.[5] As Church, we invite

---

2   Bishop Donal Murray, St John's Cathedral, Chrism Mass, Tuesday 22 March 2005.

3   'Strengthened in Holy Communion by the Body of Christ, they then manifest in a concrete way that unity of the people of God which is suitably signified and wondrously brought about by this most august sacrament', (*Lumen Gentium*, 2).

4   Pope Francis speaking to organisers of 2020 International Year of the Eucharist Conference. November 2019, Rome. www.ncronline.org/news/vatican/francis-chronicles/eucharist-creates-communion-world-needs-pope-says.

5   Augustine, Sermon 272 on the Eucharist: 'Be what you see and receive what you are'; available online: earlychurchtexts.com/public/augustine_sermon_272_eucharist.htm.

people to recognise themselves as united in one body:

> Vatican II emphasised how this communion is expressed and nourished in the Church through Word and Sacrament, beginning with Baptism and finding its summit and source in the celebration of the Eucharist.[6]

We speak of the nourishment available to the faith community when we gather as one, of the call to create an inclusive eucharistic community as a witness to the world that Christ lives here, with us, in us and through us. We have created pastoral structures[7] based on this theology, from national to parish level, employing staff and volunteers in monumental efforts to create a church that mirrors this vision of Church as *Communio*.[8]

In practice, however, our operative theology of Eucharist in Irish parish life has adapted the *structures* faster than the *understanding* of *Communio*. How else could most parishes in Ireland have managed to survive with almost no pastoral decision-making meetings for six months, or have been so quickly and fully impressed with the newly repopularised Spiritual Communion prayer, a prayer which encourages people to pray: 'I embrace You as if You were already (in my heart)'.[9] Any teaching that Jesus is not present by Baptism, that we are not in fact a temple of the Holy Spirit, and that Christ would only be truly present if one were physically receiving the sacrament of Eucharist, is unhelpful.

However unintentional, the swift dropping of 'us' for 'me', is revealing. Are 'my rights' more important than the Common Good,

---

6   Episcopal Commission for Pastoral Renewal and Adult Faith Development, *Parish Pastoral Councils A Framework for Developing Diocesan Norms and Parish Guidelines* (Dublin: Veritas, 2007) 10.
7   Structures for inclusion like the Commission for Pastoral Renewal and Adult Faith Development which created the excellent *Living Communion: Vision and Practice for Parish Pastoral Councils in Ireland* (Dublin: Veritas, 2011) were central, and relied heavily on baptised volunteers in every parish/diocese co-operating in creating Parish Pastoral Councils (PPCs) and other necessary frameworks to advance the vision of a parish that was not primarily a structure or a building but 'a family of God, a fellowship afire with a unifying spirit' (LG, 28).
8   Bishop Walter Kasper, 'The Church as *Communio*,' New Blackfriars 74 (May 1993) 232–244.
9   'An Act of Spiritual Communion', www.ewtn.com/catholicism/devotions/act-of-spiritual-communion-339. 'Since I cannot at this moment receive You sacramentally, come at least spiritually into my heart. I embrace You as if You were already there and unite myself wholly to You'.

or being part of the Body of Christ? Was this a missed opportunity to develop parishioners' personal relationship with God, family prayer, or sense of service as ministry? Why were our strongest visible pronouncements as Church, (in mainstream media) focused almost solely on the deprivation of public Mass, as if it were the sole true source of nearness to Jesus Christ?

How we celebrated Eucharist in these times
It has been instructive to consider how we have been celebrating Eucharist since March 2020, and what this reveals about intentional and unintentional understandings of Eucharist and of ourselves as a eucharistic community in this pandemic.

When churches closed suddenly in March, there was a deep genuine sadness among both clergy and parishioners. Some of this was a breaking of the daily routine, which is very human and understandable; but much of the sadness came from a genuine love and appreciation for daily Eucharist, particularly as experienced by many morning Mass-goers who now found themselves in the category of 'cocooned' (over 70 years).

As a Church our initial response was for cocooned clergy to serve cocooned Mass-goers, by offering online daily celebration of the Eucharist from home, church or chapel. I initially found myself charmed and consoled by the simplicity of praying with my priest uncle and other far-flung clergy friends as they celebrated Eucharist online in their homes. It was often the first time in my life that I had sat and listened to their thoughts on the gospel over days and weeks. I briefly wondered about a Zoom Mass rather than a webcam, as an inclusive way to hear fresh voices and prayers from the faithful, but a friend who offered precisely this was told by a lay participant in feedback that there was no need for Zoom as 'getting Mass' was enough: people really didn't need to feel part of it!

So daily Mass became the primary visible task of clergy in Ireland during COVID-19 and talk of gathering parish pastoral councils, liturgy groups or others in social justice ministry together to reflect on the mission of the parish was, in general, not deemed to be possible or necessary in this unusual moment.[10]

At the same time local GAA clubs and community organisations formed ad-hoc committees, with county champions organised to consider how vulnerable people might be fed, supported, and connected with. While clergy joined some of these teams in an individual capacity, only a few parishes or dioceses engaged in a visible way at this coalface. In truth, many parishioners were heavily involved in this amazing service, and the loss here was not that we had the experience, but perhaps that we missed the meaning.

While noble and well received, this focus on daily Mass ultimately did not reflect the full reality of the parish in that moment, nor of those whom the whole parish (not just the clergy) were called to serve.

This is not an indictment of those good men who did what they could – it is the reality of how we reacted and prioritised in an unprecedented once-in-a-lifetime crisis: we did some things as before, dropped other things, and found a balance for the rest based on our energy and needs.

What needs to be emphasised again is that the work of parish is not just the work of its clergy, and indeed that the role of parish clergy is to draw out the gifts of the whole parish, not simply to serve all. It is perfectly reasonable that diocesan clergy could not do everything – I suggest that it is not their job to do so. It is their job to lead, to discern and to invite all to make the best use of their God-given talents in this time. [11]

As Easter 2020 crept up on us, and we came to terms with the longevity of this absence from each other and a church building, we found ourselves considering how Easter symbols and rituals could be shared via screens and as families at home.

Webcams that hadn't been used regularly were brushed off and Facebook Live was discovered by clergy now cocooned, who were

---

10 Huge credit goes to any parish that did Zoom as a Parish Pastoral Council before requests for volunteer cleaners began.
11 Bishop Donal Murray, St John's Cathedral, Chrism Mass, Tuesday 22 March 2005.

looking for an accessible way to support and stay connected with parishioners. While this was an immediate answer to a short-term issue, many parishes found themselves using new, broken or challenging technology with little or no reflection on its purpose or ultimate aim. Everyone did their best, but it is worth noting that the focus was on how to get church out to people, not on how to dialogue or to listen. The instinct was to preach, to reach out. Pope Francis's call, however, was to go out, to open the doors.

Holy Week 2020 provided a telling opportunity to look at how liturgy was being celebrated in Ireland. The sheer number of ceremonies on offer was dazzling – but the liturgy itself was often not so dazzling, as many key moments were out of shot of the webcam or hard to hear. I found myself wishing for one, well prepared, well delivered service attended by thousands with some non-clerical voices or faces to remind me that Eucharist was about including the baptised, not just occupying the ordained. We have the technology to deliver this – but the operative factor still seemed to be that every local church should be open and seen to 'do something'. Yet liturgy is not just about doing something, but about being who we are.

We are one Body.

So, a very human focus on doing rather than being, drove us into the arms of much needed technology, but perhaps that 'doing' avoided the very silence and unease that was so frightening for so many, and that they sought the Church's help to cope with. What would it look like if we stopped 'doing' and reflected on who we were and are being now?

Reflections from the road

In this time of change, how did we reflect on ministry and on how we might minister now? Did we consciously choose what liturgy was appropriate in this moment, or reflect on how the community was engaging? Did parish pastoral councils or liturgy groups meet (online) to reflect on how public prayer – especially Eucharist – was chosen, prepared and led as a parish?

There was some thinking happening. I was very struck, for instance, by how many citizens embraced the RTÉ / State invite to light candles on Easter Saturday night, and the almost complete lack of a public linking that to the Paschal Fire. This was not the job of the State to do, but ours. We generally kept that conversation only to those who tuned into 'our' Paschal Fire on 'our' channels, that night.

I can recall attending only a few alternatives to Mass in those March–May weeks in 2020 – some morning prayer with mainly female religious communities, and lovely evening prayer with the Taizé community, which was a balm for many. The majority of parishes focused on Masses and Holy Week ceremonies as the thing that people desired most. Yet every parish with a Facebook page could have invited a local couple to lead the Rosary as night prayer. A few parishes with pastoral workers offered family prayer, but that surely wasn't widely promoted or encouraged as normal when it might have been an ideal time to help parents develop a routine of night prayer with their children. And what happened to the apparently vital Liturgy of the Word or of the Hours when Father no longer wanted a day off in the week because he was cocooned and had nothing else to do? Where was the pastoral leadership in these decisions and what was our focus saying about our pastoral priorities?

If Eucharist is a call to be the Body of Christ in the community rather than a personal path to heaven, surely some connection between the huge volunteer efforts happening and the community at prayer was central. Yet the focus remained stoutly on the cocooned and comforting them in their distress. A noble aim, but one that removed the capability of those over 70 to be a prayerful force for good in their community – a ministry team praying for volunteers, not just for the sick or for the avoidance of illness.

A way ahead?
Now, I don't think every parish should have thought of everything – that would be cruel hindsight! Instead I am suggesting that the role of leadership is to step back from the busy activity and to think

for the group that is itself too busy and worried to reflect. In that reflection these questions might emerge:

- What do parishioners (not just Mass-goers) most need currently? What are the primary concerns, fears, griefs, joys, hopes and dreams of the baptised in our area? What are the concerns of the wider community too, that we are called to serve?
- What are the gospel values that underpin our understanding of ourselves as Catholic – the calling we are committed to, the resources and energy God has given us in this time?
- How can we respond in thoughts, words and deeds at this time so that we are alive in our faith and a witness to God's love in this place?

I suggest that we could and can respond prayerfully, practically and peaceably in this time.

Responding prayerfully
The greatest need of our time is peace and hope. People are mithered. Ordinary assurances and plans are in pieces, and the old normal has collapsed. This is painful for an independent free adult like myself or many of my priest friends; but it's absolutely terrifying for a parent or carer for elderly parents, or a business owner employing twenty local people.

In response, there has been a huge uptake in meditation, yoga, mindfulness, walking in nature, stillness – indeed any activity that helps us to get out of our head and into a calmer body. One of the gifts we have as Christians is two thousand years of development of such calmness. As a friend commented – we have been jolted into monasticism, and the Church is full of people with skills on surviving and thriving in monastic life.

- How can parishes and cathedrals move beyond offering only one form of liturgy and offer regular, Scripture-based, still moments of peace and hope in daily life?
- How might the promotion of short, good quality meditation-

reflections online (like Sacred Space) reach far more people than 10am Mass? Why is that not a priority and what is prioritised over it?

- Funerals have been a huge source of loss and hurt for many – while we cannot change COVID-realities, could we offer a regular online prayer or liturgy for all those bereaved each week / month?
- Many searching for mindfulness find the teachings of the Desert Fathers very helpful – could dioceses or larger parishes offer Christian mindfulness or similar support?

Responding practically
Connecting the reality of life with our Christian faith is easier than we might think. While it is important that we remember our ill and dying in our prayers, for some this avoids the challenge of solidarity with our fellow citizens. Can we, as parish, find creative ways to respond to the current challenge?

- Connect faith and life in concrete ways … identify local projects to include in our liturgy and prayer. Not as announcements, but as examples used in homilies, as suggestions for charity, and in our prayers.
- Share hope. Show signs of resurrection! Create a community garden in the parish lawn, and invite people to plant and enjoy daffodils blooming in spring. Engage with the local community to create joyful moments together.
- Insist that parishioners are not an audience, but disciples, by actively creating ministry opportunities for all. … can we develop a prayer ministry for those cocooning, for instance, who might be invited to individually pray for anyone preparing for a sacrament? This might be a wonderful phone network for a Baptism or Visitation team to coordinate.
- Engage with local community development workers, GAA clubs or a St Vincent de Paul group so as to be aware of what's available and needed. Recognise that every parish is a fantastic channel of communication and use every parish communication (website, social media, emails, letters) as an opportunity to share local sup-

port available to those who need financial help, mental health support, food or company or clothing or lifts. Be a visible witness to love.

Responding peacefully
While we may experience ourselves as trapped, closed down or unable to do all that we might like, we are, in fact, in a mission moment. We are in the moment when all the things that seemed important and necessary are floating away. We all find ourselves looking for what matters amidst what remains. In this time, we are, in fact, disciples who can live from faith and be witnesses to something more.

A parish's temptation in these weeks might be 'how will we get people back in?', but that ship has sailed. We have taught people well to stay in the back row. At one time that back row was men waiting outside church before Mass started, then it was an expanding gap between those 'doing something' up front and the rest in the porch, then it was watching the Pope in the Phoenix Park on TV, and now it is daily Mass on TV, and for many, there is a sense that very little is lost in this movement.

What we need now is a new theology of Eucharist, a new conversation about what matters and how we pray together as Christians. Nothing less will suffice. This is not evangelism or a catechism for those outside of ourselves in order that 'they' come back to 'us'. This is a new theology for clergy and Mass-goers, for ministers and servants, so that we might recognise what we have fallen into in this time – and how we might move from occupying clergy into honest fresh celebrations of Eucharist, and of life, together. To quote Pope Francis:

> Just like the disciples on the road to Emmaus, the Lord will also accompany us in future through His word and through the breaking of bread in the Eucharist. And He will say to us: 'Do not be afraid! For I have overcome death.'[12]

---

12 Devin Watkins, 'Pope pens preface to book on hope in the COVID-19 pandemic', *Vatican News*, 28/07/20.

If we begin from a place of 'how will we get enough people for Confirmation preparation?' rather than 'how have people experienced life in these times?', we risk forcing people to be square pegs in round holes, and experience tells us they will just refuse to be forced into being so anymore.

The invitation into being what we want rather than what they need anymore is to give up the old maps. Trust that God, who is acting through this time, will not let the Church die, but is offering a new opportunity to imagine who we are and how we might be now. We will emerge totally new from this – how we emerge will be a measure of how much we fight against reality and how much we cooperate and listen for God's plan.

Responding prayerfully, practically and peacefully offers a path for disciples to engage with parish as a community in which to live our faith. It will not keep us visibly busy; it will be difficult and slow. However, it is the real stuff of faith and it will build up the Body of Christ which is who we are and who we deeply need to recognise ourselves as now.

Questions for Reflection and Discussion

1. Have I reflected honestly about my Covid-experience as a person of faith? Have I shared that reflection with anyone else? Where was God in this past year, for me?

2. How could we, as parish, reflect on where God is in this time, and how we might support each other practically and spiritually?

3. April is a time for the garden – what is blooming in our community? what needs to be nurtured? What blooms would most benefit all our parishioners, young and old and how can we plant and tend together?

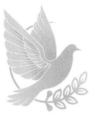

The Final Rupture?
COVID-19 and Popular Religious
Practice in Ireland

Salvador Ryan

*I*t was a few days before Christmas 1987 and a close friend and neighbour of ours had arrived at our doorstep laden down with gifts. I still remember my mother opening up the large box which contained some exquisitely patterned dinnerware. Nothing as fancy as this had ever crossed the threshold of our kitchen. There were also some chocolates, the customary tin of biscuits (most probably Afternoon Tea) and a carefully chosen Christmas card. But, wait, there was something else; a smaller box; and whatever it contained felt a little heavy in a twelve-year-old's hands. As fingers scrambled to tear away the festive sellotape and unseal the flaps, we found that the little box contained a bundle of softback books, bound together with string.

They seemed to be part of a set. Laid out on the table, their titles revealed themselves to us: *All About the Angels*; *The Wonders of the Holy Name*; *Read me or Rue it*; *How to be Happy, How to be Holy*; *The Secret of Confession*; *An Easy Way to be a Saint*, and *How to Avoid Purgatory* – okay, Christmas gifts were a little different in mid-1980s' Ireland! They were all by the same author, E.D.M. (*Enfant de Marie*), aka Fr Paul O'Sullivan, OP (1871–1958), a Kerry man who spent much of his religious life in Lisbon where he established a Catholic press with a view to releasing short catechetical and devotional works to reignite the faith in his adopted land.[1] They would also make their way back to Ireland. In 1987 they were still being sold in the St Martin Apostolate in Parnell Square, Dublin, site of the famous 'Moving Crib'. The shiny-covered books, which reflected the fairy lights of the Christmas tree under which they sat, were immensely appealing to the eye, and I soon found myself picking up the largest; it was a nice shade of yellow as far as I can remember; and it promised to teach the following: *How to be Happy, How to be Holy.* I opened the cover and flicked through the first few pages …

When future historians come to write the history of Irish Catholicism in the twenty-first century, it is very likely the year 2020 will serve as a marker of profound religious change. It will take its place along with 1850 (the date of the Synod of Thurles, but more importantly, shorthand for the beginning of the so-called 'Devotional Revolution' which transformed religious practice in Ireland); 1932 (the Eucharistic Congress, which gave the fledgling state a world stage on which to exhibit its Catholic identity); 1979 (the visit of Pope John Paul II, which numerous commentators today regard as Irish Catholicism's swansong, even if many contemporaries never guessed it); 1992 (the breaking of the Bishop Eamon Casey story, which seemed to precipitate a torrent of revelations of double-standards, abuse and cover-up over the succeeding decades); 2011 (the year in which an Irish Taoiseach, Enda Kenny, delivered a fiery speech of unprecedented candour, denouncing the 'dysfunction, disconnection, elitism and narcissism' of the Vatican in what he claimed was an attempt to frustrate the Cloyne inquiry); and, finally, the visit of Pope Francis to Ireland in 2018 which, despite his being one of the most popular popes of recent memory, failed to ignite the enthusiasm of Irish Catholics, thousands of whom chose, instead, to stay away.

---

1   For a short introduction to O'Sullivan see Thomas Casey, 'Father Paul O'Sullivan, OP, EDM (1871–1958)', in Salvador Ryan (ed.), *Treasures of Irish Christianity, volume III: To the Ends of the Earth* (Dublin: Veritas, 2015), 199–201.

These are defining dates in the history of Irish Catholicism; but 2020 may very well be the most defining date of them all. Despite lacking the triumphalism of 1932, the showmanship of 1979, the shock of 1992, or, indeed, the raw passion of 2011, it may yet be that the events of 2020 have the most far-reaching consequences for religious practice in Ireland.

But 2020 was far in the future for a twelve-year-old boy holding a book written by a long-dead Kerry Dominican in the days leading up to Christmas 1987. What he was about to discover was that every single day that he woke up was an opportunity for him to join in the most noble enterprise that one could imagine: a universal apostolate of prayer that had nothing less than the whole world in its sights – not to mention the realm of the dead who had long since passed from this world. And all one had to do was to sanctify the bits and pieces of everyday life by turning them into countless small offerings to God, and thus to take on board the line of scripture which was positioned underneath the author's name on the book's title page: 'Pray without ceasing' (1 Thess 5:17). According to O'Sullivan, the key to achieving this was to begin well upon waking in the morning. Here's what he had to say about the prayer that was once a staple of Catholic daily prayer, the 'Morning Offering':

> This act is short but we should say it with full deliberation. It is of the highest importance, for it transforms every act of the day, every work, every suffering into an act of love we can thus perform! What immense graces we shall receive! What glory we shall give to God! And if we do not make this short act, what thousands of graces we lose every day. But can there be any doubt of this fact? None whatever.[2]

While the assuredness of the assertion was very much of its time in such spiritual writing, when one gets past the style, O'Sullivan

2 Fr Paul O'Sullivan, OP (E.D.M), *How to be Happy, How to be Holy* (first published Lisbon, 1943; repr. Charlotte, NC: Tan Books, 1989), chapter 1.

was simply emphasising how natural it can be to sanctify the various elements of one's day by consciously turning each of our acts towards God. He continues, a few lines further on, by encouraging his readers to repeat this offering in a few words at various points during the day:

> For instance, when one is walking, 'O my God, I wish that every step be an act of love for you'. What is to prevent us saying a few times every day, 'O my God, every word I say I wish to be an act of love for you'. When writing, we may pause for a moment and say to God: 'My God, every word I write I wish to be an act of love for you'. Some ladies, when sewing, have the pious custom of saying, 'O my Jesus, I wish that every stitch I give be an act of love for you'.[3]

It is all too easy today to smile at such pious practices; however, to do so would be to miss the underlying thrust of such devotional exercises: a healthy spirituality does not compartmentalise communication with God by confining it to places that are considered to be 'sacred', while relegating all other areas of our life to the realm of the profane. That is hardly incarnational theology. By contrast, what O'Sullivan was proposing, in his homespun style, was that there are no areas of our life which cannot or should not be brought to God in prayer, and the recitation of short aspirations (as they were known then) were one of the means by which one did so. As a twelve-year-old boy, I could not have described his approach in those terms. But the lesson wasn't lost on me.

The spirituality found in the works of Fr Paul O'Sullivan is emblematic of a period in Irish Catholicism, often closely identified with the decades before the Second Vatican Council, but also post-dating it, in which a plethora of pious exercises and devotions were part-and-parcel of everyday life. Yes, there were the Forty Hours, Benediction, Corpus Christi processions, May altars, visiting

3   Ibid.

the seven churches on Holy Thursday, First Friday devotions, novenas to various saints, or for the Holy Souls, men's and ladies' retreats,
parish missions, pilgrimages to Knock, Croagh Patrick, and Lough
Derg, and, later, diocesan pilgrimages to international shrines such as
Lourdes. Sodalities and confraternities abounded – so much so that it
was often remarked that a person could be expected to be asked in a
job interview not whether he or she was a member of a confraternity,
but precisely which confraternity he or she was a member of. Most of
these practices were communal in nature, often bringing large numbers of people together in a shared religious experience.[4] However,
these will not be the primary focus of our attention here. Rather, I
would like to move from the large-scale practices found in the church
and the street to those that took place behind the closed (but rarely
locked) doors of family homes.

Devotion is first nurtured in domesticity; it's where practice
becomes habit, and habit becomes a way of life. For all its deficien-
cies (and there were many), pre-conciliar Irish Catholicism was not
confined to the experience of the Sunday liturgy. Catholic family life
was subsumed in religious iconography and one's day was punctuated
by domestic ritual. There were morning and night prayers, and the
Angelus bell called people to pause in prayer at noon and six o'clock.
The customary grace before meals was encouraged or, at the very least
in some households, a hastily made Sign of the Cross. And then there
was the recitation of the Rosary, a staple practice in a great many
Catholic households across the country, although by no means all.

Even when we weren't actively praying, we were encountering the
sacred at every turn, whether that was the brown scapular that one
wore around the neck; or the Miraculous Medal; or the feel of the
rosary beads in one's pocket; or the dipping in and out of the holy
water font in our comings and goings; or the habitual sprinkling of
some excess holy water to ease the suffering of the 'poor souls in

---

4   For an excellent local study of these expressions of devotion, see Síle de Chléir, *Popular*
    Catholicism in 20ᵗʰ Century Ireland: Locality, Identity and Culture (London: Bloomsbury,
    2017).

Purgatory'. It was also in our everyday speech: 'God save all here'; 'God bless'; 'God be good to him / her'; 'God bless us and save us'; 'God between us and all harm'; 'Holy Mother of God'; 'Jesus, Mary and Joseph'; or, indeed, 'Merciful hour!' (a favourite of the late broadcaster Gay Byrne). There were prayers to St Joseph for a happy death, prayers to our Guardian Angels for protection, to St Anthony for lost items, to St Jude for hopeless cases and, if you were a Pioneer (which many were), a daily pledge to the Sacred Heart to abstain from all intoxicating drinks in reparation for the sin of drunkenness.

Most of the time, often unconsciously rather than consciously, we lived and breathed a Catholicism that was interwoven with everyday life. And while that culture of Catholicism is often associated with a pre-Second-Vatican-Council Church, it certainly didn't cease to be in the 1960s. Indeed, the remnants, although becoming increasingly fragmented by this stage, were still to be found in the 1980s' rural Ireland in which I grew up. This was a time when busloads of adult pilgrims to Marian grottoes could, with childlike confidence, petition the Virgin Mary to favour their day with a pleasant surprise:

> O Mary my mother and Our Lady of Surprises, what a happy joy you caused the wedding guests when you asked your Divine Son to work the miracle of water into wine; what a happy surprise for them since they thought the wine had run dry! I, too, Mary, love surprises, and as your child I ask you to favour me with one today. I ask this only because you are my ever-caring Mother, Amen.

This is not a sophisticated prayer; but it is a heartfelt one. And it asks not for a great miracle of healing or the transformation of a difficult situation, but simply for a gentle in-breaking of divine favour to temporarily lift the humdrumness of everyday living. Some might regard such a prayer with scorn. Why bother the Mother of God with such a trivial request? And yet prayers such as this affirm that there is nothing so trivial in one's daily life that cannot be presented for God's blessing. That easy, familiar relationship with the heavenly court was a characteristic of native Irish spirituality for centuries; it's what has ensured that one can still sometimes hear recited, in the 'trimmings' of the rosary, colloquial prayers such as the following: 'O Mary, my mother, help me! You can't say you can't because you're his mother; you won't say you won't because you are my mother; so you will, won't you?', or, more pithily (to St Thérèse of Lisieux), 'Holy Flower, show your power, in this hour!' without anyone breaking a smirk.

The variegated tapestry of popular devotions that was a feature of pre-conciliar Catholicism afforded the laity a degree of agency in their spiritual lives at a time when they were largely excluded from full and active participation in the liturgy. Indeed, the reform of the liturgy which culminated in the Second Vatican Council's *Sacrosanctum Concilium* (SC) stated that 'In the restoration and promotion of the sacred liturgy, this full and active participation by all the people is the aim to be considered before all else; for it is the primary and indispensable source from which the faithful are to derive the true Christian spirit' (SC, 14) and that 'to promote active participation, the people should be encouraged to take part by means of acclamations, responses, psalmody, antiphons, and songs, as well as by actions, gestures and bodily attitudes' (SC, 30). No longer was it deemed fitting for attendees at Mass to quietly finger their beads, or leaf through their prayer books in the pew, while the priest got on with what was regarded as being his duty alone.

The liturgical reforms of the Second Vatican Council provided a necessary corrective to what was now often dismissed as an overly privatised piety of the past, and one practised by a people who were, until then, largely alienated from the richness of the Church's liturgical life. For many of the liturgical reformers of the twentieth century, the problem with many popular devotions was that they provided a very poor substitute for active participation in the Church's liturgical and sacramental life. And although *Sacrosanctum Concilium* noted that 'Popular devotions of the Christian people are to be highly commended, provided they accord with the laws and norms of the Church' (SC, 13), this need to correct a long-standing imbalance in the religious practice of Catholics would (in conjunction with wider changes in culture and society) unwittingly create a perfect storm of suspicion, and sometimes denigration, of many elements of popular piety which would come to be grudgingly tolerated by some and counted as risible relics of a theologically impoverished past by others.

The reaction against excessive legalism and scrupulosity of the past (for instance, could you approach the altar rail for Holy Communion if you had inadvertently swallowed some rain water while cycling to Mass, thus potentially breaking the fast?) led also to an inevitable loosening of devotional belts. Was it really that big a deal to miss out on reciting one's morning and evening prayers? To tuck into one's dinner before saying the customary Grace? To dash out the door without dipping one's fingers in the holy water? To pass a church or graveyard without blessing oneself? To neglect to wear some sacramental such as a scapular or medal? Surely it would be embarrassing in this day and age to suddenly fall silent and recite the Angelus when in company if you heard that church bell ring? Was God really that bothered about these little things; these rituals that one often performed by rote, even mindlessly? Was it not better to fully devote one's attention to these matters in their proper place; their designated devotional area? And increasingly, as the decades wore on, and the family Rosary now inconveniently clashed with Coronation Street (which began to win the ratings contest), that designated devotional area increasingly became a designated liturgical one: attendance at Sunday Mass. This, at least, was the one time in the week into which a person could plough his or her pious energies. And, after all, didn't the Second Vatican Council in its Dogmatic Constitution *Lumen Gentium* (1964) state that the Eucharist is 'the fount and apex of the Christian life' (LG, 11). Surely this was a case of choosing the better part? And yet very soon it became the only part.

There's no doubt whatsoever that the increased participation of the laity in the liturgical life of the Church post-Second-Vatican-

Council was a very good thing. And numbers of Irish Catholics attending Mass remained remarkably high, in comparison to other European countries, until relatively recently. The problem was that other forms of devotional life began to wane, whether those in church such as Benediction or various novena devotions; or at home such as morning and night prayers, the recitation of the family rosary, and the use of sacramentals. As a result, the single weekly point of contact with the expression of faith came to be one's attendance at Saturday evening or Sunday Mass. And despite the increased participation that the reforms of the Second Vatican Council brought in, this was nonetheless a liturgical celebration that couldn't take place without the priest. A lay person might proclaim the Word in the readings; might lead the congregation in song; might assist in the distribution of Holy Communion as a Eucharistic minister; but, ultimately, it is always the priest who presides.

Over time, then, despite the widespread caricature of the pre-Second-Vatican-Council Church being a clerically-dominated one (and the laity rendered mute in being asked to simply 'pray, pay and obey'), it's actually the post-Second-Vatican-Council Church which has witnessed a silencing of the laity, in particular in the domestic setting, albeit one that it never intended. Cara Delay, in her recent study of Irish women and Catholicism from 1850 to 1950, has highlighted the often-under-emphasised agency of women during this particular period. She remarks that 'the home would continue to be a feminised devotional space right through the middle of the twentieth century. When they led their families in prayer Irish women … also established their authority within the holy household'.[5]

With the gradual disappearance of the vestiges of domestic devotion in more recent years, however, the role of the laity in general, and women in particular, in both structuring and leading religious practice in the home also dissipated. Along with that came a reinforcement of the idea that it was predominantly the priest's role to

---

5   Cara Delay, *Irish Women and the Creation of Modern Catholicism, 1850–1950* (Manchester: Manchester University Press, 2019) 151.

lead the people in communal prayer. I remember some years ago my own parish priest received a call on his mobile when he hadn't arrived on time to say the rosary at the house of a deceased parishioner:

'It's nine o'clock, Father,' one of the neighbours explained over the phone.

'Yes, I'm sorry,' he replied, 'I've just got delayed; I'll be there as soon as I can.'

'But we're waiting for you to say the Rosary,' the neighbour continued.

A little exasperated, the priest replied: 'Are there no other Catholics present that could recite it in the meantime?'

The priest in question was a great enabler of lay participation at all levels and simply couldn't understand how a large group of parishioners needing to recite a familiar prayer could experience such a state of paralysis in the absence of a priest. Questions such as these are the inevitable consequence of a long process of disengagement with domestic devotion, something which has left us far more dependent on our clergy than we ought to be in an era when the universal call to holiness is particularly emphasised. One simply cannot imagine this situation arising in the pre-conciliar period in a domestic setting. As Eamon Duffy notes, 'Our predecessors often got the theological formulae wrong, as we in our turn will no doubt do: but they knew how to pray. We can still learn from them'.[6]

In March 2015, in preparation for the Limerick Diocesan Synod of the following year, I was invited to give a talk to some delegates, which included a reflection on some of the contemporary challenges that the Synod might address. Having delivered an overview of the history of Irish Catholicism as it evolved over the centuries, I clearly remember asking the following question:

> Would we miss it (Christianity and the practice of our faith) if it was all gone away in the morning? The answer

6   Eamon Duffy, *Faith of our Fathers* (London: Continuum, 2004) 28.

may be alarming. In fact, experience tells us that many people who walk away simply don't. And yet they should; we should. If one decides to leave a sumptuous table and to abstain from its delectable fare, surely one must starve, or at the very least suffer malnourishment? But so often that is not the case. Why? Could it, perhaps, be that the food wasn't so sumptuous after all? Or was very badly cooked![7]

Little did I realise at the time that five years later so many of us would experience precisely that: it 'all going away' very suddenly. But it didn't all go away, surely, did it? All that happened was that many of us were deprived of the opportunity to attend Mass as usual on Sundays. But my question is: with the removal of attendance at Mass from my weekly religious practice, what was left?

By 2020, for many Irish Catholics (but by no means all), Sunday Mass *was* the last vestige of religious practice. If, in the decades following the Second Vatican Council, for all sorts of cultural, societal and even religious reasons, we had participated in a religious rupture, a large scale jettisoning of devotional practice in the home, and there was a much reduced menu of non-liturgical communal devotions on offer besides, then the Sunday Mass inevitably became that which many still clung to, even if (at a time of a flood of clerical scandals) it was by their very fingernails.

And then COVID-19 hits. Very soon there is a lockdown and we can no longer attend the liturgy in person in our churches. The clergy in our parishes respond as swiftly and as generously as they can in transitioning to the provision of streamed Masses online. The national broadcaster also responds unstintingly in allowing viewers to get their daily Mass. Many parishes enthusiastically report encouraging figures tuning in. However, there are also large numbers of Mass-goers who don't. It's just not the same. It's now been a few months and there are many who haven't attended Mass since;

---

7   Some of the notes from that talk can be found here: www.synod2016.com/resources-for-delegates/the-history-of-synods-in-ireland-by-dr-salvador-ryan.

and given the fact that the sky hasn't fallen in, many within this category may never return. Might 2020 be the year that marks the final rupture in the history of Irish Catholicism? Could a global pandemic finally do for some, especially those still barely clinging on, what almost three decades of scandalous revelations failed to do, like a swift December breeze sweeping away the last of the autumnal leaves?

What is for sure is that the first rupture has not helped us in our coping with the prospect of a possible second. A healthy Christian life cannot sustain itself by simply leap-frogging from Sunday to Sunday without anything in between. By doing that, it is simply bone without cartilage. To become truly COVID-proof, we need both. What we celebrate in the Sunday liturgy should naturally overflow into our weekly living, our communal worship and our domestic religious practice, becoming, for us, a seamless garment. Domestic devotion offers us an opportunity to embed in our daily lives rituals that will carry memory and meaning for the long haul, and may, at least in part, sustain us in times of eucharistic famine. In this time of COVID-19, with no clear end yet in view, we may need to return to the site of that first rupture to find the clues necessary to avoid a second.

Questions for Reflection and Discussion

1. Recall some religious practice from your childhood: what are your memories of your experience of it at the time?
2. What function did sacramentals – and the tangible – play in popular religious devotion in the past, such as the wearing of a crucifix, religious medals or scapulars, the use of holy water, and the lighting of blessed candles? What part do these (or sacramentals like them) play in the lives of Christians to this day?
3. How has the experience of being deprived of the opportunity to attend the Liturgy of the Eucharist these past months been? Are

there things you have really missed by not attending? Or maybe not? Has it caused you to view the Eucharist differently in any way?

4. What has your experience been of viewing the celebration of the Eucharist online or on television if, indeed, you have done so? If you do tune in, why do you consider it important to do so?

5. If you were to begin one daily religious practice in your home, what would it be and why?

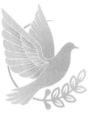

Singing the Lord's Song
in a Strange Land
(or How to Pray When Our World Falls to Pieces)

Jessie Rogers

*H*ow do we pray in the midst of a pandemic that drags on and on and scrambles every aspect of life? In this situation the 'Help, Lord!' cries that arise naturally in response to a sudden crisis are not enough. Our prayer has time to develop and deepen. But do we know how to pray those more expansive prayers? If our prayer seems hollow or God seems distant, it could be that there is a disconnect between what we say and how we feel or what we are experiencing.

The psalms mark out various paths in the terrain of faith, with different start- and end-points. The people of God who came before us addressed God from myriad circumstances, and Scripture bequeaths some of their wisdom to us. The prayers that are preserved in the Book of Psalms are Spirit-inspired gifts that can help us to walk our own authentic journeys. The psalms do not only provide *words* to pray; they also model the *pattern* of prayer for different situations.

In this chapter, I look at two such psalm-prayers, reflecting on their shape as much as on their content, highlighting the movement and the shifts that occur in them. This provides a window onto the spirituality that they embody, not as a state so much as a process which can draw us along so that we do not get stuck. The steps may be surprising, but they are time-honoured and proven stepping-stones for living faith in a chaotic world. Psalm 137 is a prayer for when the earth under our feet has shifted, while Psalm 77 puts words on the seasickness of finding that our very sense of God has shifted. Both are prayed from places of deeply uncomfortable newness.

The journey from 'there' to 'here'

> By the rivers of Babylon –
> there we sat down and there we wept
> when we remembered Zion.
> On the willows there
> we hung up our harps.
> For there our captors
> asked us for songs,
> and our tormentors asked for mirth, saying,
> 'Sing us one of the songs of Zion!'
>
> How could we sing the Lord's song
> in a foreign land? (Ps 137:1–4)

Psalm 137 is a song of exile. It originates in Babylonia where the people of God had been settled after being forcibly taken from their homeland. It is the prayer of a traumatised people who have seen their beloved Jerusalem, the centre of their world, utterly destroyed and who find themselves in a strange and hostile place. Their situation is akin to the Rohingya in the refugee camps in Bangladesh and is the story of millions displaced through violence and war. In the face of such loss and such grief, how can they pray? The displacement and alienation brought about due to COVID-19 and the measures put in place to contain it are a lot less brutal, but they are disorientating, confusing and wrenching nonetheless. It is a psalm that can be prayed from within any experience of 'exile' where we find ourselves ejected from the world that was 'home' into a frightening and uncomfortable place.

There are a number of stages in this psalm which plot a path into exile, a way of beginning the long hard labour of mourning for all that is lost, so that space can begin to open up for something new. It does not take the person praying all the way through to the other side of the chaos, but it does get them started on the journey. And those first steps can be the hardest to take.

The psalm begins in grief, but a grief enveloped in denial. Four times in the opening lines of the translation (but only twice in the Hebrew original), the word 'there' is used. Grammarians call this the farther demonstrative, in contrast to 'here' which is the nearer demonstrative. This gives the impression that this prayer is not actually prayed by the rivers of Babylon, but looks at the experience from a distance. That word 'there' hints strongly at denial, a distancing, an initial refusal or inability to be present in this new, strange space. The prayer begins in a place of emotional and imaginative distancing from present experience. Although they are in exile, they were still dwelling in the old world which had ended. The journey still had to be taken from 'there' to 'here'. Physically they may have been in Babylonia, but their souls and their hearts had to follow their bodies into exile, to acknowledge and to accept this new reality. Being thrust into exile is something that happened to them, but entering the experience of exile is a journey they themselves need to take. The task of entering exile is captured in the poignant question: 'How could we sing the Lord's song in a foreign land?' At this point in the process the answer seems to be: 'It is impossible.'

> If I forget you, O Jerusalem,
> let my right hand wither!
> Let my tongue cling to the roof of my mouth,
> if I do not remember you,
> if I do not set Jerusalem
> above my highest joy. (Ps 137:5–6)

All the emotional energy in this psalm is directed to the past, and to the old place. That is where God was known, and it seems that if that is let go of, then the connection with God will also be lost. Worship in the new space seems to be impossible except as a commitment to the old. The harps fall silent. There is only the shame of failure, of helplessness before those who mock. How indeed can the songs of Zion be sung, the songs that celebrate God's greatness and God's special care for God's people? Zion is in ruins, destroyed. The prayer has already suggested the project for the future – singing the Lord's song in this new place – but that is still only known as an impossibility. All that can be done at this stage is a commitment to remember. There is real fear, aggressively couched in self-cursing, that forgetfulness might cause them to lose everything. The past and memory is the anchor in the storm.

We know that, with the passage of time, God's people did learn to sing the Lord's song in the new place. The two seemingly irreconcilable elements – remembering Jerusalem and settling into the present situation – would come together in a faithful exilic community. If they stayed with remembering Jerusalem as it was, refusing the imaginative and theological journey into exile, they would have remained stuck. But if they forgot Jerusalem, they would have assimilated completely to the culture in which they now found themselves, and lost their identity as God's people. They are going to have to remember Jerusalem *and* sing the Lord's song in a foreign land. The memory that threatens to paralyse them will become energising. Over the course of time, they will learn how to embrace the new in a way that is faithful to the old.

But they are not there yet. The new song has not yet taken shape. This psalm is a prayer for that moment when the ending is grieved, and the beginning is not yet discerned. It is not a moral lesson about how one *ought* to feel, or an exemplar of what things look and feel like once the tension is resolved. It is a prayer to give expression to this anguished moment of entering into exile, an invitation and a pattern for entering deeply into it, because, if God's people do not enter deeply into exile, they will not be able to move forward and beyond this moment. It is a prayer that does not look back on the crisis from a safe distance, but cries out from the thick of it. The psalm does give the next step, and it is a shocking one, so much so that the Church has decided not to offer it in her public prayer. Most of the following verses are not heard in the Liturgy of the Word and are excised from the Liturgy of the Hours:

> Remember, O Lord, against the Edomites
> the day of Jerusalem's fall,
> how they said, 'Tear it down! Tear it down!
> Down to its foundations!'
> O daughter Babylon, you devastator!
> Happy shall they be who pay you back
> what you have done to us!
> Happy shall they be who take your little ones
> and dash them against the rock! (Ps 137:7–9)

The pain and violence experienced in the destruction of Jerusalem leads into a cry of rage and plea for God's vengeance, both against the neighbours who took advantage of Jerusalem's plight and the perpetrators of the evils of the destruction, that those who inflicted such atrocities would become the recipients of the same. The cry is that the violence be returned on their own head, in a way which pierces their own humanity. At this point Christian commentators often jump in to say that we cannot pray like this, writing these words off as sub-Christian.[1] I believe, though, that there are times when this is the only way that people can pray authentically and honestly before God.

Unlike mothers in war-torn countries, I have not watched my children being violated and slaughtered before my helpless gaze, but I am sure that the cry of rage and grief and even desire for revenge

---

1   Erich Zenger, *A God of Vengeance? Understanding the Psalms of Divine Wrath* (Louisville, KY: Westminster John Knox Press, 1996) provides a masterful exploration and critique of Christian antipathy to psalms like this, and suggests how their wise use can enrich Christian worship.

in that moment would be an expression of God-given human love and connection arising from the depths of the soul. If we do not give expression to our grief, which often comes out in the first place as anger, it will destroy us or shut us down. This is not an advocacy of violence so much as a cry to God that justice be done. In giving us these horrifying words which, please God, we will never need in order to voice our own anguish, the psalm gives us permission to take all our emotions, raw and unfiltered, into prayer.

This emotional honesty, this giving expression to the grief, even as hate-filled anger, is key to being able to move into and through this stage. It is not the end-point to which we are moving, but it is the next step. In prayer before God, we can plumb the depths of our reactions and give them all to God, who does not judge them. Only on the other side of this uncomfortable honesty will we be able to find a new song to sing in the strange land. The journey from 'there' to 'here', to being able to find God in the now, passes through this vulnerable space of giving vent to what is already there within us.

How can this psalm help us to pray in a time of COVID-19? Psalm 137 gives us powerful images of grieving; it invites us to pour out our hearts in all their complexity to God, to begin that journey into exile. The fact that this psalm is part of Scripture is a powerful affirmation that we can bring everything to God in prayer. The journey to life and healing does not happen as a prerequisite to acceptable prayer; the transformation happens *in* prayer. We come as we are. This is a prayer to pray early in the process, a prayer to utter in the dark; and it does not take us all the way through to the light. Not every prayer is a prayer of arrival. Some, like this one, are prayers for the intermediate stages.

'God has changed'

Psalm 77 is another psalm that expresses difficult emotions. It begins as a typical prayer of lament. There are many such prayers in the Book of Psalms, pleas for God to hear, to respond and to save in a time of crisis. But Psalm 77 is distinctive in that it addresses a crisis of faith in the midst of the external crisis. It models prayer in the teeth of a potential loss of faith in a good and familiar God.

My Bible adds a title for this psalm: 'God's Mighty Deeds Recalled.' That makes it sound like a straightforward celebration of God's story with God's people, but it is more complicated than that. It will take a journey of several stages that Walter Brueggemann calls the turn from the self to God.[2]

> I cry aloud to God,
> aloud to God, that he may hear me.
> In the day of my trouble I seek the Lord;
> in the night my hand is stretched out without wearying;
> my soul refuses to be comforted.
> I think of God, and I moan;
> I meditate, and my spirit faints.
> You keep my eyelids from closing;
> I am so troubled that I cannot speak.
> I consider the days of old,
> and remember the years of long ago.
> I commune with my heart in the night;
> I meditate and search my spirit. (Ps 77:1–6)

Although these words are addressed to God, the focus is still overwhelmingly on the praying person's own actions and attempts to move God to respond. The psalm begins where one needs to start when engulfed by a crisis: in the now and with the self. 'I' do this, and 'I' do that. God is the object of this seeking and pleading. In fact, the only thing that God is said to do in these opening verses is to rob the complainant of sleep! The present difficulty fills the horizon. The crisis leads to introspection and a sense of being cut off from God. God is spoken *about*, not *to*. The past is the longed-for country that

---

2   Walter Brueggemann, 'The "Turn" from Self to God: Psalm 77', chapter 5 in *Virus as a Summons to Faith. Biblical Reflections in a Time of Loss, Grief and Uncertainty* (Eugene, OR: Cascade Books, 2020). My reading of Psalm 77 is strongly indebted to this masterful interpretation.

is no longer accessible. All one has are memories of God, a cherished tradition, and deafening silence from heaven.

But then the prayer does switch the focus onto God in a series of rhetorical questions. The God who is known, the God of the covenant who keeps promises and rescues God's people – what has happened to that God? The only way to interpret what is happening, in terms of past understanding of God, is that God has become harsh and forgetful, that God's mercy and grace have ceased. These words mourn the passing of a simpler and safer time, and a simpler and safer God.

> 'Will the Lord spurn forever,
> and never again be favourable?
> Has his steadfast love ceased forever?
> Are his promises at an end for all time?
> Has God forgotten to be gracious?
> Has he in anger shut up his compassion?'
> And I say, 'It is my grief
> that the right hand of the Most High has changed.' (Ps 77:7–10)

The person praying reaches a point of naming their grief: the power of the Lord to intervene, to keep God's people safe, to answer prayers and do miracles, all of that seems to have changed. The sure and stable sense of who God is, and what God can be relied upon to do, has been shattered. Is this a loss of faith, or is it an opening to new faith for new times? In the present moment, it can feel like the former. But, because the doubt and disappointment is expressed in prayer, the way is open for the Spirit to gently nudge toward new and deeper faith.

This psalm invites the candid admission of disappointment in God, and then offers a next step. Now God is spoken to directly. The past is still in view, but more as *God's* story. The old stories that nourished and anchored a secure and confident faith are still there, they are still true, but they are beginning to be reframed to take account of God's freedom. The mystery of God comes into view and eclipses a smaller image of God as the strong and safe guarantor of our own life and worldview. God is committed to God's people, but for God's good purposes, not our little ones. And it is precisely God's freedom that is our hope. God will not be dragged down to serve our little agendas, but by God's grace we are caught up in God's great plan.

> I will call to mind the deeds of the Lord;
> I will remember your wonders of old.
> I will meditate on all your work,
> and muse on your mighty deeds.
> Your way, O God, is holy.
> What god is so great as our God?
> You are the God who works wonders;
> you have displayed your might among the peoples.
> With your strong arm you redeemed your people,
> the descendants of Jacob and Joseph.
>
> When the waters saw you, O God,
> when the waters saw you, they were afraid;
> the very deep trembled.
> The clouds poured out water;
> the skies thundered;
> your arrows flashed on every side.
> The crash of your thunder was in the whirlwind;
> your lightnings lit up the world;
> the earth trembled and shook.
>
> Your way was through the sea,
> your path, through the mighty waters;
> yet your footprints were unseen.
> You led your people like a flock
> by the hand of Moses and Aaron. (Ps 77:11–20)

The God whose power can be seen in creation is the God of the

Exodus, the God who redeems God's people, the God and Father of our Lord Jesus Christ. But this prayer nudges us beyond remembering the story of salvation in a way which tries to tie God to a formula for how to act. The footprints of the redeeming God are unseen, even as God's redemptive activity cannot be doubted. The psalm ends abruptly here, in the past, but with the assurance of God's leading. To quote Walter Brueggemann, 'Nothing has been resolved, but everything has been recontextualised'. The way of faith is not carved in stone, but plotted out by God's unseen footprints.

The journey reflected in this psalm is from the disorientation of a certain faith that has been shipwrecked on the confusing events of life, through disillusionment with God, to a reorientation toward a deeper faith that knows less yet trusts more. It is a dangerous journey, but even here God will lead us.

How can we pray in a time of COVID-19? These psalms invite us to pray honest, unfiltered prayers. In times when we push up against our limits, we are tempted to take the path of denial and numbness, with our heads in the sand and eyes closed. But prayers that come from that space will be hollow and meaningless. Or we may want to turn to prayer as a kind of magic, to find the incantations that will make God do something or change the world. But that makes both God and prayer too small; it denies God's freedom and it refuses the gift that God is offering us in this strange space. However, when we recognise that our prayer is itself a part of the journey, when we accept the invitation of these psalms to bring our deepest fears, angers and doubts into prayer, we open ourselves to the God who can lead us through this strange terrain. With the Spirit's help, we learn to sing God's song in a foreign land.

Questions for Reflection and Discussion

1. How does the psalmist's experience of going into exile resonate with your experience of the COVID-19 crisis?
2. Has the pandemic, with all the changes it has brought, caused you to question God and God's commitment to you?
3. Are you comfortable with expressing your desires and feelings in prayer, even the 'bad' or unacceptable ones? Or do you think there are things that we are not allowed to say to God?
4. Do you sense an invitation to pray differently in the light of Psalms 137 and 77?

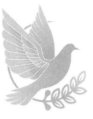

Exile and Sabbath: Scriptural Models for a Time of Pandemic

Jeremy Corley

'*B*y the rivers of Babylon, there we sat and wept' (Ps 137:1).[1] After the pandemic struck, we entered into something of the grief experienced by the Jewish exiles deported to Babylon in the sixth century BCE. During 2020, we wept because of the lives lost to a disease for which there was no known cure at that time. We wept because of the number of frail and elderly patients who died after catching COVID-19.

We grieved because we lost some beloved members of our own community to the virus – perhaps even members of our own family or friends. We grieved for families denied a normal funeral for a loved one who had passed away. We grieved because some COVID-19 victims were buried with only a few simple graveside prayers, attended only by the closest relatives.

We wept because the hospitals were overwhelmed with patients. We wept because so many sick people were in intensive care units and emergency treatment rooms. And we wept because relatives could not visit sick members of the family in hospital,

---

1   This is one of the lament psalms. See G. Brooke Lester, 'Psalms of Lament', www.bibleodyssey.org:443/passages/related-articles/psalms-of-lament.

even during their last hours of life on this earth.

And we lamented for the wider disruption to society, affecting almost everyone. We lamented for all the people who suddenly lost their jobs, with no idea when they would be able to find work again. We lamented for families confined to inadequate accommodation. We lamented for victims of domestic abuse, trapped in the same house as the abuser.

We also felt sorry for ourselves, because our limitations became very visible. We felt sorry because the virus reminded us forcefully of our human mortality: 'Dust you are, and to dust you shall return' (Gen 3:19). We felt sorry because the pandemic reminded us that for each of us, our time on earth is limited.

And we lamented the disruption to our own lives. We lamented because we could no longer go to work as usual. We lamented because our normal lives had suddenly been turned completely upside down. We lamented because for many of us, with hardly any warning, all or some of our livelihood was taken away.

We also felt sad because we were frequently confined to home, unable to visit friends and relatives. We felt sad because grandparents were no longer able to see grandchildren. We felt sad because often the only way we could speak to family and friends was through a phone or a computer screen.

We grieved the disappearance of our familiar world and lamented the loss of our normal lives. We lamented all the family and parish events cancelled. We lamented the disruption caused by the postponement of many First Holy Communions, Confirmations and weddings. We lamented all the sports events cancelled and long-awaited matches that had to be deferred. We lamented the many cultural events postponed or suspended – festivals, meetings and concerts. And we lamented because we were no longer able to have Mass with our parish community.

Because of the pandemic, we have felt exiled from our normal lives. We have been exiled from members of our family and our groups of friends. We have been exiled from our workplaces. We have been exiled from the 'temple' of our parish churches, which were often left locked for many long weeks.

Sometimes the lockdown felt like a prison experience for the whole community, restricting our freedom to go where we liked. Whereas previously we could choose to travel anywhere throughout the country, or abroad, we have at times been limited to a certain area specified by the government. While we have recognised that these restrictions have been for our own good, they have still sometimes left us feeling hemmed in.

These restrictions have shown us that we are ultimately not in total control of our lives. We have faced limitations in what we can do and where we can go. We have needed to follow government guidelines. We have been dependent on others telling us what to do. We have come to see clearly how much we rely on those who supply us with food and other essential goods, as well as those who provide for our health.

Ultimately, we recognise once again that we are dependent on God. Our lives are vulnerable, because there is now a hidden enemy – sometimes an unseen killer – present in the form of the virus. News of the rollout of the vaccine from the end of 2020 brought us hope. Meanwhile, all we have been able to do is take sensible precautions, and then commit our lives and our health to God's will.

During this time of 'exile', we have been able to look at the Scriptures for help in making some sense of what has happened to us. We can see how the scriptural authors came to understand their experience of being deported into exile in the strange land of Babylon.[2] We have been able to share their feelings of being alienated from all that was familiar, being forced to adapt reluctantly to new circumstances.

The exile in the sixth century BCE was such a terrible event for the people of Israel, because the Jerusalem temple had been the centre of their worship. Moreover, the religion was so closely linked to living in the Promised Land, that losing the land led some of them

---

2   Martien A. Halvorson-Taylor, 'Exile in the Hebrew Bible', www.bibleodyssey.org:443/places/related-articles/exile-in-the-hebrew-bible.

to begin questioning their faith. If God had previously chosen and saved them, why had he allowed this disaster to happen? In a comparable way, the pandemic has called into question many of our certainties – sometimes leading to great distress and even despair. Just as the people of Israel had to relearn their relationship with God through the trauma of exile, so we have had to do something similar during these difficult months.

One scriptural interpretation of the exile taught the Israelites that the land needed to make up its Sabbaths, which had been missed during many previous years. In a sense, the land required time for rest and replenishment. After Jerusalem had fallen to the enemy, the Book of Chronicles offers this interpretation of the deportation to Babylon: 'King Nebuchadnezzar took into exile in Babylon those who had escaped from the sword, until the land had made up for its Sabbaths. All the days that it lay desolate, the land kept Sabbath' (2 Chr 36:20–21).

The author of Chronicles here refers to the seventh-day pattern of Sabbath rest stipulated in the Ten Commandments (Exod 20:8–11).[3] After six days of labouring, each Israelite was commanded to rest on the seventh day. In an unusual ecological move, however, the author of Chronicles speaks, not of the resting of human beings, but of rest for the land itself.

For the biblical author, the sinfulness of the people of Israel caused them to be taken into exile in Babylon, leaving the land free to enjoy its Sabbath rest. For us today, the shutdown because of the virus often felt like a home exile, while we have been away from our normal workplaces. Yet like the Jewish Sabbath, this time has perhaps allowed us the space to reflect on our lives and rediscover what is truly important for us.

The Book of Chronicles, written in hindsight after the exile was over, echoes the stark warning previously given to the people of Israel

---

3   Catherine E. Bonesho, 'Sabbath', www.bibleodyssey.org:443/passages/related-articles/ sabbath. See also William P. Brown, 'Ten Commandments (Exod 20)', www.bibleodyssey. org:443/en/passages/main-articles/the-decalogue.

in the Book of Leviticus. The ancient text warned that if God's people went astray, he would remove them from the Promised Land and let the ground remain fallow: 'As long as the land lies desolate, it shall have the rest it did not have on your Sabbaths when you were living on it' (Lev 26:35).

During the Babylonian exile (587–538 BCE) the Jewish people were away from their country, until the land enjoyed its Sabbaths – the Sabbaths it had not experienced during the previous years. For us, while the farmland has continued to be cultivated, the towns and cities have often experienced a notable Sabbath. Restaurants and bars have often been closed, streets have been empty, and many workplaces have been shut down for several months.

The first creation story in the Book of Genesis describes God creating the world in six days, and then taking his Sabbath rest. 'On the seventh day God finished the work that he had done, and he rested on the seventh day' (Gen 2:2). However, until the pandemic reached us early in 2020, our society tended to operate 24/7, without taking time for resting. Perhaps we have tended to overlook at our peril the wisdom that God offered us in the Scriptures.

During the lockdowns, people had to stay at home. Instead of the mad daily rush of work and leisure, many people suddenly found themselves with more time on their hands. There was time to think and reflect, time to appreciate nature, and hopefully time for prayer. There was also much more time for parents to be with their young children. As the restrictions began to ease after the first wave of the virus in 2020, parents would more often go out for a family walk with their young children.

During the first lockdown in early 2020, it sometimes felt as though nature had pressed the pause button on our human lives. In normally busy cities across the world – Los Angeles, Beijing and Delhi – blue skies once again became visible, without the pall of soot and smog. Fish were once again seen in the canals of Venice.

Just as the Babylonian exile and the destruction of the Jerusalem temple meant that the Jewish people were away from their traditional forms of worship, so during the lockdown the church buildings were closed and there were no public Masses. People needed to rediscover personal and family forms of prayer. Many watched livestreamed Masses that were available.

Nevertheless, there has also been a definite sense of loss. For several months during 2020, people were unable to receive Holy Communion, even at Easter. There has been the loss of the sense of belonging, as people have been unable to join the faith community physically for worship.

As we look through the Scriptures, we find that time and time again, hardships and difficulties became occasions to offer prayers for God's mercy – prayers that were so often answered. When the Israelites in the desert suffered punishment from lethal snakebites after complaining against God, they cried out (Num 21:5–9). Then God told Moses to set up a bronze serpent, so that anyone looking at it would live. In St John's Gospel, this bronze serpent lifted up on a pole becomes a symbol of the crucified Christ who saves us (John 3:14–15).

Later, David's pride in numbering the people of Israel was seen as leading to punishment by a severe plague (2 Sam 24:1–25). In response to David's pleading for the people, God answered his prayer by bringing an end to the pestilence. The very site of this incident became the location where the Jerusalem temple was subsequently built.

Then, at the dedication of the temple, David's son Solomon offered this prayer for the people of Israel: 'If they sin against you, and they are carried away captive to the land of the enemy, and if they come to their senses in the land of their captivity, and repent, and plead with you, then hear their prayer, and forgive your people who have sinned against you' (1 Kings 8:46–50).

King Solomon's prayer at the dedication of the temple looks ahead to a time when the people may end up in exile after being forgetful and neglectful of God. He urges God to be forgiving if the people acknowledge their previous faults. During this time of shutdown, we have perhaps realised that, even if we are not great sinners, we have sometimes forgotten what is most significant in life. But in these months of enforced idleness, we have hopefully been able to rediscover God and turn back to him.

At a later time of national crisis, the prophet Joel called the people to gather together physically in heartfelt prayer: 'Call a solemn assembly. Gather the people. Between the vestibule and the altar let the priests, the ministers of the Lord, weep. Let them say: Spare your people, O Lord' (Joel 2:15–17). Although physical gatherings have been limited during the COVID-19 pandemic, we have been able to unite spiritually in offering the same plea to God: 'Spare your people, O Lord.' Faced with a disease for which no medical cure was originally available, we have been asking God to spare us and all his people. And recently, we have rejoiced in the rollout of several vaccines against the virus.

The wise teacher Sirach reminds us that serving God does not always make life easy, but that we need to be ready for testing. Yet he also offers us this encouragement: 'Has anyone persevered in the fear of the Lord and been forsaken? Or has anyone called upon him and been neglected?' (Sir 2:10). Examples from Scripture show us the divine mercy: 'The Lord is compassionate and merciful. He forgives sins and saves in time of distress' (Sir 2:11).

God's compassion for the people of Israel is clearly evident in the unexpected ending of the Babylonian exile. After two generations in a foreign land, God marvellously sent the Israelites a deliverer in the form of the Persian king Cyrus.[4] Following his conquest of Babylon, he allowed the various deported and exiled peoples to return to their homelands, including the people of Israel.

The conclusion of the Book of Chronicles reports the decree issued by King Cyrus: 'The Lord, the God of heaven, has given me all the kingdoms of the earth, and he has commissioned me to build him a temple at Jerusalem, which is in Judah. Whoever is among you of

---

4   Lisbeth S. Fried, 'Cyrus the Messiah', http://bibleodyssey.org/en/people/related-articles/cyrus-the-messiah.

all his people, may the Lord his God be with him! Let him go up' (2 Chr 36:23). We can imagine the joy of the exiled Jews finally allowed to return home and rebuild the temple.[5]

To be sure, when the Jewish exiles came back to their homeland, they still faced difficulties. There were many financial hardships for the returning community. In that context, the prophet Haggai urged them to rebuild the Jerusalem temple, and then God would bless them – as indeed happened (Hag 1:5–13).

The fact that God so often heard the prayers of the Israelites in times of distress gives us hope that after the severe testing of the pandemic, he will once again restore us and enable us to rebuild our lives. We rejoice that several vaccines have been developed and introduced to combat the virus, and we hope that public health will be restored widely.

Hopefully we will have learnt from our experiences. Perhaps we have discovered a greater appreciation for our families and all those who share our lives. Perhaps we have relearnt the value of family time – not doing anything in particular, but just being present with those who share our household.

Maybe we have also learnt the value of the health workers caring for patients, day in and day out. Maybe we have learnt greater respect for the carers looking after vulnerable people, without receiving a great financial reward. Maybe we have discovered the value of the key workers who keep our lives safe and supplied.

Possibly we have learnt that we do not need to be busy nonstop with work and social events, travel and bustle. Possibly we have discovered the wisdom of the Jewish Sabbath, that gives time and space for rest and reflection. Possibly we have learnt to appreciate stillness and quiet. Perhaps we have developed more patience for silence and waiting.

Perhaps also we have learnt to appreciate the small things in life: a hot meal on a cold day, a cool drink on a hot day, a flower budding,

5   Tamara Cohn Eskenazi, 'Destruction and Reconstruction of the Temple', www.bibleodyssey. org:443/places/related-articles/destruction-and-reconstruction-of-the-temple.

a tree producing its leaves, a kind word or gesture. Perhaps we have gained a deeper appreciation of creation in all its beauty and wonder: the sunshine and clouds, the rain falling on a dry lawn or field, the wind moving through the trees, the birds gathering twigs to build a nest, a rose bush coming into bloom, or the view of a distant mountain or hill.

Maybe we have learnt to treasure the presence of God within us, both in good times and in bad: 'Be still and know that I am God' (Ps 46:10). Maybe we have learnt to trust more in God who tells us: 'Do not be afraid' (Jn 6:20). Maybe we have learnt to accept the reassuring words of Julian of Norwich: 'All shall be well, and all shall be well, and all manner of thing shall be well.'[6]

Perhaps we have again learnt to treasure the assurance given in Psalm 23: 'The Lord is my shepherd; I shall not want... Even though I walk through the darkest valley, I fear no evil, for you are with me' (Ps 23:1, 4). In this time when there has been so much fear, we have been invited to trust in divine providence. We need not fear evil, because God is with us, even in the darkest valley. If Jesus has walked through suffering, even to the point of death, he is with us throughout our lives. Let us trust him to deliver us.

Questions for Reflection and Discussion

1. How far have we experienced the pandemic as a time of exile, like the Jewish exiles in Babylon?
2. How has our experience of prayer changed during the months of COVID-19 restrictions?
3. Have we rediscovered some Sabbath values during the pandemic?
4. In the past months of COVID-19, which other Scripture passages have helped you?

---

6   Mahri Leonard-Fleckman, 'Julian of Norwich believed "All will be well." Would she say so today?' *America Magazine* 223/2 (August 2020), www.americamagazine.org/faith/2020/06/24/julian-norwich-believed-all-will-be-well-would-she-say-so-today.

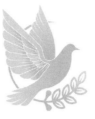

Theodicy:
Where is God in COVID-19?

Noel O'Sullivan

'As flies to wanton boys are we to the gods;
they kill us for their sport.'
(Shakespeare, *King Lear,* Act IV, scene I, lines 37–38)

'From the beginning till now the entire creation, as we
know, has been groaning in one great act of giving birth;
and not only creation, but all of us who possess the first-
fruits of the Spirit, we too groan inwardly as we wait for
our bodies to be set free.'
(St Paul to the Romans 8:22–23)

*M*uch has been written about COVID-19, most of it
excellent. So what is different about this chapter? Here
we are situating the pandemic in the wider context of suffering and
evil which has always beleaguered the human condition. How can
one find meaning living through a world-wide threat to our very
existence? Is it possible to believe in a loving and all-powerful God as
we wade our way through this trauma?

At the outset it is important to clarify our approach. I prefer to
speak of the mystery of evil and suffering, rather than designate it

as a problem. The latter implies that there is a solution. 'Mystery' suggests that the issue is bigger than any of us; more far-reaching even than humanity itself. So our task is precise: to explore ways in which we can live with the mystery of evil and suffering; in this case the pandemic, COVID-19. In our exploration we will outline the main currents of the human response to the vulnerability of life, culminating in Christ's own encounter with suffering and evil. I will begin with two statements from the street:

1. God has felt let down by the world and that is why he sent us the coronavirus.
2. There is a holy woman who had a vision in which she was told that coronavirus is the work of the devil.

These are two 'street statements' I heard in March 2020 from people who firmly believed what they were saying. The first saw COVID-19 as a punishment from God for a world that had betrayed him; the second was convinced of its satanic provenance. Both interlocutors had solved the problem of evil; they knew its cause! Since then I have heard many variants of those two statements.

In a crisis like this pandemic we clamour for answers and all too often we jump to facile conclusions. Somehow, having an answer or explanation makes pain more bearable. Of course, these two statements say more about those who utter them than about the veracity or otherwise of what they state. The first presents an image of a vengeful God while the second understands the world as susceptible to the unfettered activity of the devil. In this, the latter shows a residue of Manichaeism, on which I shall comment presently.

Few have remained untouched by the fear and dread which have gripped the world since the start of the pandemic. Among those affected were the millions who were diagnosed positive for COVID-19, not knowing if they would survive. Their situation was further exacerbated as those who were hospitalised were deprived of the personal presence of family. The attendant issues of job losses and financial strain brought national economies to their knees and, as always, the poor suffered most. And then there were the other illnesses that went untreated and undiagnosed for months because of the fear of infection. Many have experienced extreme suffering, either personally or vicariously, due to the pandemic.

Here we intend to try to make sense of living through this crisis, drawing on the philosophical and theological tradition which has wrestled with suffering and evil throughout history. The focus will be on a response inspired by faith in Christ but, first of all, we will explore briefly how humanity in general responds to the pain of existence. Some questions are apposite by way of an initial engagement with the issue. Has our Christian faith made a difference? Have we begged God to save us from this deadly virus? Do we feel he is listening? Or have we dismissed religious faith as so much 'pie in the sky' which is of no earthly use in the face of a real life-and-death situation?

From time immemorial, different peoples and cultures have attempted to make sense of suffering and evil in the world. They have tried to reconcile their experience of pain and desolation with their belief in a loving, all-powerful God. The area of study which explores this issue is called 'theodicy'. It will be the umbrella under which we will tease out a religious response to COVID-19. Although the term 'theodicy' is attributed to Gottfried Leibniz (1646–1716), the issue it attempts to treat is as old as humanity. In his introduction to the second edition of his classic work, *Evil and the God of Love*, John Hick summed up the problematic of his book and we can take it as the problematic of this chapter. He wrote:

> The sheer crushing weight of the pains suffered by men, women and children, and also by the lower animals, including that inflicted by human greed, cruelty and malevolence, undoubtedly constitutes the biggest obstacle that there is to belief in an all-powerful and loving Creator.[1]

1   John Hick, *Evil and the God of Love* (Basingstoke: Palgrave Macmillan, [1966] 2010), x.

This is our subject. Can suffering and evil be reconciled with belief in God? Where is God in our COVID-19 world? And what is this God like?

We can readily distinguish between two kinds of suffering; moral suffering caused by human beings is the first; the second category is what is inflicted on the world by natural disasters. Moral evil is manifest in domestic violence, sexual exploitation, blatantly unjust political and economic systems. Knowing who is responsible for our suffering does not diminish our pain. But natural disasters, like the 2004 Indian Ocean tsunami, evoke a sense of hopelessness and make belief in God challenging at best, impossible at worst. The lines uttered by Edgar in *King Lear* when he meets his father, Gloucester, whose eyes have been gouged out, suggest that we are the playthings of malevolent gods or God: 'As flies to wanton boys are we to the gods; they kill us for their sport' (*King Lear,* Act IV, scene I, lines 37–38). Here we are asking: Is there an alternative to this despair?

A creaky creation?

Cosmological theories (as to how the world began) have offered solutions to the problem of suffering and evil by proffering the view that we live in a faulty creation, which has its provenance in an imperfect or weak god. One such theory is found in the Enuma Elish epic of Mesopotamia which dates back to the seventeenth century BCE. It describes the beginning of the world in terms of conflict. Marduk emerges as the most powerful of the gods and destroys the goddess Tiamat. Out of her dismembered body the world is formed. With this nefarious beginning the world is inevitably bad. It contrasts so much with the accounts of creation in Genesis where the world emerges effortlessly from the word of God and creation is inherently good. The Enuma Elish epic leaves us in no doubt but that evil has its source in creation itself.

A major impetus was given to a negative view of creation by the movement known as Gnosticism. Its beginnings are unclear, but it certainly was a significant force in Jewish and early Christian thought. Gnosticism is based on the belief that the world was created by a lesser god which thereby explains the origin of evil. The name 'gnostic' derives from the Greek word *gnosis*, meaning knowledge. Gnosticism proposes salvation through knowledge.

Characteristic of the Gnostic teaching was the distinction between the Demiurge or 'creator god' and the Supreme, remote and unknowable Divine Being. From the latter, the Demiurge was derived by a series of emanations or 'aeons'. He it was who, through some mischance or fall among the higher aeons, was the immediate source of creation, which was therefore imperfect and antagonistic to what was truly spiritual. Creation, in a Gnostic perspective, is basically evil; the human person is a prisoner in a body incapable of salvation. Gnosticism is anti-historical because the human person has no possibility of progress towards salvation. Only the elect can enter the *Pleroma* or fullness of existence.[2] Human freedom does not exist. But into the constitution of some people there had entered a seed or spark of a divine spiritual substance, and through 'gnosis' and the rites associated with it this spiritual element might be rescued from its evil material environment and assured of a return to its home in the Divine Being. Such people were designated the 'spiritual' (*pneumatikoi*), while others were merely 'fleshy' or 'material' (*sarkikoi*) and were doomed to perdition. According to this view, the function of Christ was to come as the emissary of the supreme God, bringing 'gnosis'. As a Divine Being, he neither assumed a properly human body nor died, but either temporarily inhabited a human being, Jesus, or assumed a merely phantasmal human appearance.

The negative anthropology emanating from Gnosticism resulted in attitudes which were anti-body and, effectively, anti-human, with unfortunate consequences for spirituality and the possibility of living an integrated human life. Closely associated with this philosophy was Manichaeism which had as one of its devotees a young St Augustine before his conversion to Christianity. Its founder, Mani

---

2   *Pleroma* in the New Testament is used to refer to the fact that the fullness of divinity is to be found only in Christ (Col 2:9).

(215–276 CE), explained evil in his teaching that there were two equal principles, good and evil, warring against each other. In this perspective God does not have ultimate control as God has to contend with the powerful force of evil. As I suggested earlier, the second 'street statement', that the Coronavirus is the work of the devil, falls into this category. As Christians, we need to exclude the possibility of COVID-19 having its origin in an evil source which is outside the control of a loving God.

Reality check on a Panglossian solution

A search for a solution to the problem of evil and suffering was accelerated in the seventeenth and eighteenth centuries, propelled by a new confidence in the rationalism of the Enlightenment period. Gottfried Leibniz (1646-1716) published his *Essais de Théodicée sur la bonté de Dieu* (1710) in which he defended the rationality of God and creation against attacks by philosophers like Pierre Bayle (1647–1706) who claimed it was impossible to believe in a rational and omnipotent God in the face of evil in the world. Bayle supported the Manichaean solution. Leibniz counteracted that God created the 'best of all possible worlds', while obeying the laws of reason and avoiding any logical contradiction. His *Essais* is a justification of God from which the term 'theodicy' is derived; *theos* meaning 'God' and *diké* 'justice'. Evil in his system is the result of the creature's imperfection which is prior to the Fall.

Leibniz's solution was grist to the mill of Voltaire (1694–1778) in his scathing satire *Candide ou l'Optimisme* (1759). Though Voltaire believed in a rational God, he found his experience of the world contradicted the belief that this is '*le meilleur des mondes possibles*'. He was especially traumatised by the Lisbon earthquake (1755). Voltaire's famous argument for God's existence is based on the clock; if there is a clock then there must be a clockmaker. His is a deistic belief.[3]

---

3   Deism is the belief that while God created the world God has no further dealings with it. It excludes revelation and, at best, puts its faith in natural religion. In eighteenth-century France it was particularly prevalent among the Encyclopaedists.

Candide reads as an adventure novel with the eponymous character educated in the philosophy of optimism by the German philosopher Dr Pangloss. The young student is convinced by his teacher that this is indeed the best of all possible worlds despite appearances to the contrary. Through a series of adventures Candide travels the world where he is exposed to a myriad of experiences; love and disappointment, friendship and betrayal, the glamour and cruelty of war. Despite his protestations to the contrary, Candide begins to doubt that this is the best of all possible worlds. His Panglossian education does not stand up to reality because events seem to lack any moral purpose or rational pattern. These are not just world events but his own personal experience of life, especially his love for Cunégonde who ends up marrying his own best friend.

So what is the solution? Well, it is encapsulated in the immortal words with which the novel ends: '*Il faut cultiver notre jardin*' (we must tend to our garden). In other words, Candide learns that philosophical speculation does not solve the problem; the way forward is work (at least, for those able to work). We must deal with the reality we face and just get on with it. Interestingly, gardens never seemed so well manicured as in the summer of 2020!

Evil as the privation of good (Privatio Boni)

The foregoing exploration of the problem of evil and suffering, which we might globally label philosophical, is not just a preamble to a Christian theological response. The attempts of humanity to cope with the pain of existence are not to be lightly dismissed with the presumption that Christianity offers a clear and ready-made solution. We need to accept humbly that human reason, being the gift of God, can lead us a certain distance along the way to meaning. It is the same human reason which theologians use in their quest for the truth of God. The difference is that they have revelation at their disposal. But their task is not a simple one as we shall see.

St Augustine laid the foundations of a theological response to evil and suffering. He realised that the Manichaean solution of positing a principle of evil outside of God's control was untenable for a Christian. Instead, he defined evil as *privatio boni*, the privation of good. In this he was in continuity with Neo-Platonism, especially Plotinus (c. 204–270). For the latter the One (the highest level of reality) is totally good; in other words, being and goodness are synonymous. Evil, in contrast, is non-being. According to Plotinus the Supreme Being pours out his goodness into the myriad of forms in creation and when that creativity is exhausted, we are left with evil.

While agreeing that all created being is good, Augustine does not share Plotinus' view that evil is the result of an exhausted divine creativity. For Augustine the world is the result of a free choice by God; it is not the automatic outcome of self-emanation, as Plotinus believed. Evil, in Augustine's teaching, is the malfunctioning of something that is in itself good. But because everything is made out of nothing, nature is susceptible to corruption and so evil can be seen as the corruption of the good. Augustine's understanding of evil is succinctly expressed in his *Confessions*:

> I sought to know what wickedness (*iniquitas*) was, and found it was no substance, but a perverse distortion of the will away from the highest substance and towards the lowest things.[4]

In this light we may suggest that illness is yet another element of creation functioning in a way that is not in accord with its true purpose. It does not have a metaphysical existence and, of course, it was not created by God. We can see this malfunctioning too in human sinfulness and in natural disasters like earthquakes.

But much of what is loosely described as a natural disaster may have its source in human greed (or sin). The abuse of the earth, as described by Pope Francis in his encyclical letter *Laudato Si'* (2015), is causing untold suffering to the poorest of the poor as their shanty

---

4   St Augustine, *The Confessions* VII, 16, translated by Philip Burton (London: Everyman's Library, 2001).

huts are washed away by the sea. Augustine claimed that all evil is in some way the result of the misuse of free will, as illustrated in this comment from *The City of God*:

> From the bad use of free will, there originated the whole train of evil, which, with its concatenation of miseries, con-voys [*sic*] the human race from its depraved origin, as from a corrupt root, on to the destruction of the second death, which has no end, those only being excepted who are freed by the grace of God.[5]

From this perspective evil is either the direct result of the abuse of free will or the consequences that accrue from that abuse. It does not have an existence independent of human decision.

Augustine's theodicy has shaped the Christian understanding of evil and suffering in a singular way. To recap, God created a perfect world which was undermined by the sin of Adam (Genesis 3). That sin affected every human being ever since, like a contagious virus. Original Sin is the term that encapsulates this contagion. As a result all evil is the result of sin or is a punishment for sin.

However, there is a different tradition emanating from other early Christian thinkers based on a particular interpretation of human cre-ation in the image and likeness of God (Gen 1:26–27), associated with Origen and Irenaeus of Lyons especially. Created in the image (*eikon / tselem*) of God, the human person is gifted with the divine prerogatives of reason, freedom and immortality. To use the technical term, image is 'inamissible', meaning that it can never be lost; the most depraved sinner still has something of the image of God. Like-ness (*homoiosis / demuth*), according to Irenaeus, is different. He sees it as a potential given to the human person at creation which grows under grace in the course of a person's life until they 'see God face to face' and are fully transformed into God's likeness (I John 3:2).

---

5   St Augustine, *The City of God*, Book XIII, 14, translated by Marcus Dods (New York: Modern Library Edition, 1993), 423.

On the basis of this distinction between image and likeness, Irenaeus presents an understanding of creation as a developmental process. Adam and Eve in this perspective are like vulnerable children in the Garden of Eden, in need of God's mercy, rather than two perfect human beings whose sin represents a damnable revolt. Perfection is a gradual process brought about by the loving grace of God over a lifetime. God is more like an understanding parent bringing his children to maturity than a vengeful judge watching out for every wrongdoing, ready to dole out the appropriate punishment. Irenaeus's view sits more easily with an evolutionary world view which dominates modern thinking about the world and its origins.

Few have contributed more to the reconciliation of an evolutionary world view in Christianity than the French palaeontologist, Pierre Teilhard de Chardin (1881–1955). Teilhard proposed creation as an ever-increasing process of complexification, beginning with the Geosphere (the earth), moving through the Biosphere (non-human life) and reaching its highest complexity in the Noosphere when human life appears. The three stages, then, were matter or earth (*geos*), life (*bios*) and mind (*noos*). He took the process a stage further to suggest that the final unification of all things finds its completion in the Christosphere (Omega point). In this way Teilhard, the great-grandnephew of Voltaire (!), gives a Christian understanding of evolution, identifying its goal as the recapitulation of all things in Christ (Eph 1:9–10).[6]

Here we have seen two different approaches to creation which offer us two contrasting means of understanding evil and suffering. With Augustine we move from the perfection of the Garden of Eden, destroyed by the wilful sin of our 'first parents', to the sin and pain of human existence ever since. With Teilhard we enter an evolutionary world where perfection (likeness to God) is at the end (the *telos*). The process involves suffering and evil, not as punishment but as the groans of a world coming into being. The pain we experience in life is the pain of childbirth:

6 See Noel O'Sullivan, 'Striving Towards the Omega Point,' in Brendan Leahy (ed.), *Faith and the Marvelous Progress of Science* (New York: New City Press, 2014), 141–157.

From the beginning till now the entire creation, as we know, has been groaning in one great act of giving birth; and not only creation, but all of us who possess the first-fruits of the Spirit, we too groan inwardly as we wait for our bodies to be set free. (Rom 8:22–23)

The image of childbirth does not solve the 'problem' of evil and suffering, but it does reveal to us that as a 'mystery' it has meaning. Its meaning is found in the coming together of all things in Christ, the Christosphere. How can we be sure?

In Hoc Signo Vinces: *'In this sign you shall conquer'*[7]
The answer to this question lies in the life, death and resurrection of Jesus Christ. It is the paradox of death leading to life, as manifested in Christ, that paves the way for us to live through the mystery of suffering and evil. Jesus made it very clear that renunciation of self, taking up the cross and following him is the way to full life: 'Anyone who loses his life for my sake will find it' (Mt 16:25; Lk 17:33; Jn 12:25). Physical death is not a tragedy for the person who dies; it is inexorably painful for the family of course, just as it was for Mary as she stood at the foot of the cross as her Son was dying. From a faith perspective 'life is changed not ended' (*Preface for the Dead,* 1). This change comes about through seeing the face of God and being transformed definitively into God's likeness.

The Eastern Christian tradition calls this 'divinisation'; we become gods by adoption. The prospect of contracting COVID-19 and maybe dying from it sends shivers through us but that is not the worst thing that can happen to us. Jesus says as much: 'Do not be afraid of those who kill the body but cannot kill the soul' (Mt 10:28). If God allowed his Son, Jesus, to suffer and die in an ignominious crucifixion, then it is not inconceivable that he allows humanity to share in that pain.

---

7   Reference is to the Roman Emperor, Constantine, who attributed his victory at the Battle of the Milvian Bridge (311 or 312 CE) to his vision of the cross in the sky accompanied by this dictum (Eusebius, *Life of Constantine*, 38–39; 204–13).

We may feel abandoned, as did Jesus on the cross, when he cried out in the words of Psalm 22:1[21:1], 'My God, my God, why have you deserted me?' (Mt 27:46). But Jesus was not abandoned; neither are we. He was raised from the dead; we shall also be raised from the dead. For this reason we can make the words of St Paul our own:

> I shall be very happy to make my weaknesses my special boast so that the power of Christ may stay over me, and that is why I am quite content with my weaknesses, and with insults, hardships, persecutions, and the agonies I go through for Christ's sake. For it is when I am weak that I am strong. (2 Cor 12:9–10)

The challenge is to accept the paradox: death leads to life; the cross is a sign of victory. In our view this may not be the best of all possible worlds but, when considered in conjunction with the reality beyond this physical universe, we are not the playthings of the gods. Instead, we are held in the hand of God with unconditional love, despite appearances to the contrary.

Questions for Reflection and Discussion

1. To what extent have you thought about the issues raised in this chapter? The answer to this question may involve a brief summary of these issues.
2. Has the question of evil and suffering influenced your understanding of God?
3. What is your understanding of God?
4. How has the pandemic affected your religious faith and prayer life? Have you become more or less religious as a result?

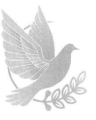

God and the Problem of Suffering: Philosophical Perspectives

Gaven Kerr

$\mathscr{C}$OVID-19 has swept across the world causing all sorts of havoc, both disrupting and ending lives. Nobody has been unaffected by COVID-19. Given the impact of the virus, people have naturally become reflective on the existential state of humanity. Amidst all our technological mastery over nature and our great success at living in the world, we have been brought low and humbled. Many people have been remaining indoors, not venturing outside, afraid to engage with family members or in normal day-to-day human activities. It is not war or some technological disaster that has brought humanity to this state, but something pertaining to nature itself.

COVID-19 has brought to the fore the fact that despite our technical advances, we are still subject to nature in a very radical way. We are not beyond nature, but a part of nature, so that when things happen in nature humanity can be affected in quite significant ways. Not only that, COVID-19 has focused our attention on the role of God in such things. God is the creator of all things; there is nothing that has its being that is not from God.[1] One would be inclined to think, then, that the current disaster has its being from God in some

---

1   For more in-depth treatment of these issues see Gaven Kerr, *Aquinas's Way to God: The Proof in* De Ente et Essentia (New York: Oxford University Press, 2015), and *Aquinas and the Metaphysics of Creation* (New York: Oxford University Press, 2019).

way. We naturally ask, and indeed are right to ask, what is God doing in bringing about the being of such suffering?

What this question highlights is the traditional problem of evil: if God exists, then evil does not exist; but evil exists, therefore God does not exist. For some, the presence of evil or suffering in the world is a strong indication that God does not exist or that God is not the wholly good and loving God that we take him to be. Indeed, St Thomas Aquinas takes the presence of evil in the world to be a significant objection to God's existence, one that he proceeds to answer.[2] I would like to address this problem in the current chapter.

Before proceeding, I want to set aside a philosophical issue pertaining to the problem of evil.[3] I have stated above that everything has its being from God; what I mean here is that every *thing* has its being from God. Sometimes we use the term 'thing' to refer to substantial entities, such as humans, trees, and rocks; but on other occasions we use the term not to refer to things, but to what are not actually things, e.g. a hole in a sock, blindness, or relations. The latter are only taken to be real because of how they affect some substantial being in some way. For example, a hole in a sock is really just a feature of the material of the sock, it itself is not a thing; blindness is a feature of how the eyes and brain function (or fail to function the way they ought) in an individual; and relations (if real) are features of how two things are constituted so as to have a bearing to each other.

From a philosophical perspective, God gives being to real substantial things, and the things that have their being can have all sorts of features pertaining to them. Crucially, in creating things, God co-creates all these various features, but it is the real substance itself that God creates, not directly its various features.[4] The latter entails that if God is all good and loving, then his creation of the substance itself is good and undertaken out of love, but that does not mean that various features of it are not lacking in goodness in some way. For

2   Aquinas, *Summa Theologiae* (Turin: Marietti, 1926), Ia, qu. 2, art. 3, obj. 1.
3   See my article, 'A Thomistic Response to the Problem of Evil', *Yearbook of the Irish Philosophical Society* (2011) 38–50.
4   For further details see Kerr, *Aquinas and the Metaphysics of Creation*, Chapter 5.

example, a human being is a good thing, but the blindness a human being suffers is not good. God creates the human, but he does not create the blindness; blindness is simply something that affects the human. Hence, God does not directly bring blindness into existence, or diseases which one suffers, and all other sorts of realities that affect our world. Rather, he brings into existence the things themselves for which it is good to exist; and these various other features that contribute to our suffering are dependent on the being of the thing. There is nothing evil then that God directly creates; all that he creates is good. Having said that, God certainly does know that creatures suffer, and given both his love and his omnipotence, the question is whether there is a morally sufficient reason for God's permitting such suffering.

The problem of suffering
We often take some suffering to be justified if a good enough outcome can be drawn from it. For instance, dental work is not very pleasant for most people, yet generally the benefit of having dental work done far outweighs the suffering of the work itself. Another example, eating a healthy diet and taking regular exercise is not always pleasant and sometimes can be described as a kind of suffering; but the benefit of a long and healthy life far outweighs the discomfort of forgoing foods and lifestyle choices which, whilst enjoyable, are bad for one's health. The point of these examples, and the more general point, is that suffering is redeemable against some sort of beneficial outcome – if it is worth it. The question then is whether God redeems suffering present in creation by providing some sort of beneficial outcome.[5]

To address the latter, I want to look at suffering as articulated in the Bible, particularly in the story of Abraham, discerning therein how God proposes to redeem suffering by some beneficial good that

---

5   This is indeed the crux of Aquinas's response to this issue, *Summa Theologiae*, Ia, qu. 2, art. 3, ad. 1: 'It pertains to the infinite goodness of God that he permits evil to exist and produce good out of it'. My translation.

he brings about. In this I am following Eleonore Stump's account from *Wandering in Darkness: Narrative and the Problem of Suffering*, wherein she offers an account of various suffering narratives in the Bible. Her account shows that God's concern throughout is with those who suffer and that the suffering is the means by which God offers a good wholly outweighing what the person suffering undergoes.[6]

Abraham is the father of faith (Rom 4:16–18) and a friend of God (Jas 2:23). In the Book of Genesis we see the story of Abraham as concerned with his desire for biological offspring. God promises a progeny to Abraham through his wife Sarah despite her old age.[7] But frustratingly for Abraham, God does not make good on his promise immediately; indeed, God makes the promise to Abraham on four separate occasions (Gen 12:2, Gen 15:1, Gen 17, Gen 18), the first being when he was seventy-five-years old. On each occasion as time moves on, we witness Abraham becoming more and more frustrated that God's promise has not been fulfilled. After the second promise in Genesis 15, Abraham and Sarah take matters into their own hands and use their maidservant Hagar to produce a son, Ishmael. Abraham is eighty-six when Ishmael is born, meaning a break of eleven years from God's original promise. Despite the seeming fulfilment of the promise in Ishmael, Abraham and, eventually, Sarah find out (Gen 17 & 18) that the son by whom Abraham will be a father of a great nation is not Ishmael, but will be from his wife Sarah. This son is Isaac and he is not born until Abraham is one hundred years old (Gen 21:5).

It is worth reflecting on the situation here. God asked Abraham to leave his home and family at the age of seventy-five under the promise of offspring. Abraham obeys but it takes twenty-five years for God's promise to come to pass. In the meantime, we have Ishmael,

---

6   Eleonore Stump, *Wandering in Darkness: Narrative and the Problem of Suffering* (Oxford: Clarendon Press, 2010), Part 3. Whilst this account is dependent on and inspired by Stump's, any misunderstanding or divergence from her intended point is entirely my own.

7   For ease of reference, I will use the final forms of the names for Abraham and Sarah, though they do not receive these names until the third promise in Genesis 17.

Abraham's son from Hagar. Ishmael is fourteen years old when Isaac is born, which means Abraham had another son for those fourteen years until God's promise comes to pass.

Not only has Abraham been put through a trying twenty-five years of faithfulness to God's promise, he is caught up in a tricky family situation and we see this emerge at a weaning party held for Isaac. During the party, Sarah perceives that Ishmael is mocking Isaac and demands that Abraham dismiss both Ishmael and Hagar (Gen 21:8). We read that Abraham was quite distressed by this, but God recommended that Abraham listen to Sarah – not because Sarah was right to dismiss Ishmael and Hagar (it is not clear that Ishmael did anything wrong, and there is no indication that Hagar did anything at all) but because God intends to bless Ishmael (Gen 21:11–14).

This seems to be the ideal outcome for Abraham. Ishmael and Hagar are gone at Sarah's request and God's concurrence. And so, we must ask a question that Stump pertinently raises: what were Abraham's motives here?[8] Abraham was distressed at having to dismiss a son that he had known and loved for fourteen years. Yet in following God's will he has managed to untangle a tricky family situation that has left him with his wife Sarah and the son that God promised to him. Following God's will in this instance was not exactly contrary to Abraham's interests, and it certainly straightened some tangled paths. It suited Abraham to follow God's will in this case. But given Abraham's previous restlessness with God's promise, we must ask what Abraham would do if God's will did not suit him: would he still be faithful? The latter is addressed in the very next episode, where we see God's request of Abraham to sacrifice his son Isaac.

Abraham has been through a lot at this stage. Already in old age, he has left family and home to follow God's will under the promise of a son. It took twenty-five years for God to make good on that promise, and in the aftermath, Abraham ended up banishing another son whom he had loved for fourteen years. In dismissing Ishmael, Abra-

8   Stump, *Wandering in Darkness*, 292–293.

ham followed God's will *and* it suited him to do so. But in being asked
to sacrifice Isaac, Abraham is being asked to follow God's will *and*
now it does not suit him to do so. Abraham is being asked to decide
whether he believes that God will remain faithful to his promise.
God promised him a son and that through him Abraham's descen-
dants would become a great nation. If God is faithful to that promise, then Abraham will retain his son, even though God asks him to
sacrifice him. Abraham's response is well known (Gen 22). He gets
up early in the morning, travels to the place of sacrifice, and lifts the
knife to sacrifice his son. At the crucial moment God brings things
to a halt, and a ram is sacrificed instead. When asked to follow God's
will when it does not suit him, Abraham still follows God's will.

We have seen that from the beginning Abraham was somewhat
hesitant in following God. He did not fully trust God's promises;
indeed he undertook to fulfil them by his own means through Ishmael. Abraham must be brought to a stage of maturity and trust in
the goodness of God, so that when God asks Abraham to sacrifice his
son, Abraham knows that God will still be faithful to his promise of
offspring; that even given such a sacrifice, God will not permit him
to lose his son. The years of suffering and doubt were God's means
for producing in Abraham the kind of love and trust in God that we
usually see only amongst the closest of friends and spouses. It took
God over twenty-five years to produce such character in Abraham.
As a result, Abraham not only had his son and thereby his progeny,
he became God's friend. Those twenty-five plus years produced in
Abraham a friendship with the Creator of all that is, so that as a
result Abraham came to enjoy close personal communion with God.

A major feature of Stump's account of this and other situations is
that the suffering undergone is redeemed through being brought into
a loving relationship with God. Scripture itself tells us that Abraham
is accounted not only the father of faith, but a friend of God (Rom
4:13; Isa 41:8). This gives us a clue, then, to the great good by which
God redeems all the suffering in the world. Any suffering undergone
can produce in the one suffering such a character that that person

can enter into communal friendship with God. In other words, God gives *himself* as the greater good by which all the suffering of creation is redeemed.

Trust rather than control

COVID-19 has brought us forcefully to the realisation that we are not masters over creation. Our rationality and ingenuity allow us to dominate creation. But we are not creators; we can simply take what has been created and modify it in some way. Only God is the Creator, and only God is the good itself. Whatever God creates, he creates as a manifestation of his goodness. There is nothing in creation, then, that God does not love, since all of creation is loved by God because it imitates the good that he himself is. Not only that, the goal of all creation is God itself. He is the end and perfection of all things. When it comes to rational creatures, then, the goal of our lives is the enjoyment of the goodness of God. This enjoyment will be proper to our nature as rational creatures; hence it will be a rational enjoyment of God. We can only enjoy God's goodness in a rational manner if we come to see God as he is. Hence, the goal of the life of any rational creature, is the face-to-face enjoyment of the presence of God, i.e. to enter into communal friendship with God.[9]

We are separated from God through sin. Sin turns us from the true good of God, to some lesser good that we take to be greater than the true good itself. As is well known in Christian thinking, sin is overcome through the second person of the Trinity, the Word, taking to himself a human nature and offering a satisfying atonement for sin. God's infinite love for all humanity is perfectly returned and satisfied through Christ. This in turn brings about the grace by which humans are sanctified and can enjoy the friendship of God. Through Christ God gives himself in friendship to all of humanity.

We noted in the ordeals of Abraham that God took many years to bring Abraham to a point where Abraham could trust in God's goodness. This level of friendship and trust was so deep in the end

9   For further details see Kerr, *Aquinas and the Metaphysics of Creation*, Chapter 7.

that Abraham knew he would not lose his son despite the situation that faced him. This disposition to enjoy the friendship of God was not initially present in Abraham, given his doubts about God's promise; it had to be inculcated through many patient years of suffering.

Stoics are famous for holding that we do not have control over what events will occur to us, but the only thing we can control are our reactions to those events. I want to suggest something similar in reaction to human suffering, though I don't want to go as far as the Stoics. The Stoic ideal is not to be troubled by *any* suffering; to bring oneself to such a state that nothing is troubling. But this is inhuman. We cannot but react to the suffering that COVID-19 has caused. What I want to suggest is that whilst we can recognise such suffering for what it is and mourn over it, we can see such suffering as an opportunity to grow in character like Abraham; in other words, we are affected by suffering but not constrained by it. We can see ourselves in Abraham's situation during those twenty-five years, his character slowly forming and his trust in God never being lost. When Abraham's character was fully formed, he had such trust in God and friendship with him that he knew that he would not lose his son.

Similarly, through suffering our character is slowly formed and our trust in God made deeper. Being brought into friendship with God, and having that love for God deepened through suffering, we know that God will be with us when we die so that we die in love with him.[10] The full reward of God's eternal presence, the supernatural happiness by which God himself is happy, will be the great good we come to enjoy through our friendship with God.[11] God redeems suffering by offering us himself, so that when we come to enjoy him we realise that no suffering undergone in this world is comparable to the least joy experienced with God in heaven (Rom 8:18). Accordingly, God is not absent in any human suffering, but always pres-

---

10 I am grateful to Prof. Eleanore Stump for initially suggesting this to me.
11 Dante, *The Divine Comedy: Paradiso*, Canto 33, 142–145: 'At this point high imagination failed; but already my desire and my will were being turned like a wheel, all at one speed, by the love which moves the sun and the other stars.' Translation by C. H. Sisson, *The Divine Comedy* (Manchester: Carcanet Press, 1980).

ent and inviting trust in him. This does not undo the suffering one undergoes, but it does redeem the suffering, since through it one is made a friend of God.

Questions for Reflection and Discussion

1. Consider how strong is the bond between two close friends or spouses. What prevents people from having the same bond with God?

2. We often feel very thankful for the friends that we have and how they have enriched our lives. Given that God offers himself to us in friendship, how does that enrich our lives?

3. Sometimes there are ordeals, not always physical, that we must undergo. The mere presence of a loved one during these ordeals makes them bearable. Now consider that all things exist because they are present to God drawing their existence from him; God is inescapable. With that in mind, how would we think about our suffering?

4. We know that nobody can escape death, but we can think about the matter in another way: nobody can avoid meeting God after death. With the latter in mind, how should we prepare ourselves for death?

5. Friendship requires effort, and the bonds of friendship can be loosened if friends do not regularly work on their friendship. How can we work on our friendship with God?

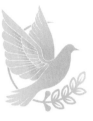

Retrieving Passion in the Pandemic: An Existential Response

Thomas G. Casey, SJ

*T*he pandemic we have been experiencing since early 2020 not only threatens our physical health; it affects us in our ways of living as well. It has altered our personal lives to varying degrees, changing everything from how we relate to each other to how we shop for groceries. It has introduced a new level of unpredictability and uncertainty into our lives. Ultimately, this crisis endangers our very existence, confronting us with our own mortality. Admittedly, there is no sense that this pandemic is going to result in the extinction of our species. However, it has led to the death of many individuals.

Whether its actual physical impact on us is large or small, this crisis is nevertheless forcing us to ask big questions. This is because many of the things we took for granted now turn out to have troubling consequences. For instance, even the simplest of gestures, such as shaking hands, entails a health risk. Another example: going to work can now potentially endanger our lives and the lives of others, so more and more people have been working from home.

To put it in slightly different words: this crisis is an existential crisis. That is because it faces us with fundamental questions about the nature and purpose of our existence. Work is a good example of how this pandemic has generated an existential crisis. Work has huge existential significance. On the one hand, it can be laborious drudgery: we need to work to survive. On the other hand, work can be rewarding and fulfilling, because when we work, we not only change things, we also change and develop ourselves. Whether positive or negative, work plays a big role in our lives.

But the COVID-19 crisis has had an impact on our working lives that we are only beginning to grasp, not least by leading to massive unemployment. Moreover, our societies are redefining what 'essential' work is, and a significant number of workers are shifting, at least temporarily, to remote work or working from home. All of these changes can have knock-on effects such as decreased levels of well-being, psychological distress, and depression. These negative effects illustrate how this pandemic is an existential crisis; since these consequences put into question our sense of who we are and what our lives are about. Any crisis that rocks us to the core is an existential crisis. It forces us to ask who we are, what we are about and where we are headed.

During this existential crisis we could benefit from receiving existentialist help. Existentialism is a concrete kind of philosophy, centred on what it means to live a truly human life, and this pandemic offers us the opportunity to ask if we are in fact living truly human lives, and if not, how we could change things for the better.

The particular existentialist thinker I would like to draw upon is Søren Kierkegaard (1813–1855). This Danish thinker, often called 'the father of existentialism', was passionate by nature. His worst nightmare was to sleepwalk through a superficial life. He was attracted by God as the Absolute, as someone absolutely incompatible with the flabby and complacent sort of religion with which too many of his contemporaries contented themselves. He did not want to get entwined in mediocre things because he was always haunted by ultimate realities.

In one sense, Søren Kierkegaard seems a figure from a past that is quite remote from our present. Born just over two hundred years ago in Copenhagen, he grew up in a world that was in many ways different to our own. Yet at the same time, many of his insights are surprisingly relevant and can prove helpful for ourselves and for our time.

But for all that, Kierkegaard does not offer the kinds of insights that necessarily make us feel better about ourselves. Although passionate, he isn't a warm and fuzzy kind of thinker. Even his name makes this clear: 'Søren' comes from the Latin and means 'severe'; while in Danish the word 'Kierkegaard' means 'cemetery'. True to his first name, Søren is severe, even toward those who, like himself, are Christians. He doesn't spare those who pretend they have faith, all the while evading the genuine demands of Christianity.

For his readers, Kierkegaard is brilliant and infuriating in equal measure. He delights in posing disconcerting and disturbing questions. He prefers to provoke rather than to pacify, to stir up rather than to soothe, to confront rather than to comfort. In addition, he often expresses his thoughts in deliberately difficult ways. He writes under so many different names that these pseudonyms make it hard to identify what his own views really are.

In this chapter, I will attempt to convey what Kierkegaard might say to us about the pandemic and its effects upon us, were he to appear in our midst today. I won't be offering a scholarly reconstruction of Kierkegaard's thought, because the object here is not complete fidelity, which according to Kierkegaard himself is in any case impossible: 'I will never be understood' as he once wrote in his diary. Instead, I will aim for a certain imaginative freedom that allows me to make his wisdom accessible to non-specialist readers.

Kierkegaard: An imaginary monologue

As a child I loved the wonderful Frederiksberg Gardens in Copenhagen, which appeared to me like an enchanted land. I continued to spend time in these gardens as an adult. I can picture myself sitting there today, almost two hundred years later, in my favourite place. As I drink from a bottle of water, I say to myself: 'all around you, people are trying their best to solve the COVID-19 crisis – doctors are run off their feet in the hospitals, scientists are working around the clock to develop better vaccines, and politicians are formulating policies for the Danish people. So many people are doing so much to solve this crisis. And what about you? What are you doing?' Here I momentarily break off my soliloquy, for I have run out of water. I stand up, take a few steps and throw the bottle into a nearby bin, before returning to the bench. At that precise moment the following thought suddenly flashes through my mind: 'You must do something, but since you are no politician or doctor or scientist, and so cannot solve this crisis, you must undertake, with the same humanitarian enthusiasm as the others, to make it even more acute.' This strange notion pleases me immensely, for when everyone cooperates to resolve a problem, there remains always the danger that it will disappear so completely that there will be no difficulties at all. Out of love for humankind, and out of despair at the awkwardness I feel in not being able to find a vaccine or offer medical assistance or show political leadership at this trying moment, I give myself the task of creating even more difficulties.[1]

And so, dear reader, whether or not you have been literally cocooned during this pandemic, my hope is to make it difficult for you to stay cocooned in complacency. When you are faced with an existential threat, your natural instinct of preservation pushes you to find ways to avoid it. One way of avoiding it is to deny that there is a crisis at all. I want to propose another path, that of facing the challenging aspects of this crisis, not in order to drive you into deeper despair, but so as to raise you up, and so that you can discover – as one of my favourite plays of all, Shakespeare's *Hamlet*, puts it, that – 'there are more things in heaven and earth…than are dreamt of in your philosophy' (Act 1, Scene 5, 167–168).

I went through my own existential crisis when I was twenty-three years old. It's not surprising that the books I later wrote had titles such as *Fear and Trembling*, *The Sickness unto Death*, and *The Concept of Anxiety*. But whatever about my written works, my personal life was already in freefall as a young adult. I was stressed and anxious. I felt emotionally overwhelmed. My mother died, and then in quick

---

1   This opening paragraph, set in Copenhagen's Frederiksberg Gardens, is loosely based on a passage from one of Kierkegaard's many pseudonymous works. See Søren Kierkegaard, *Concluding Unscientific Postscript to the Philosophical Fragments*, edited and translated with an introduction and notes by Howard and Edna Hong, (Princeton: Princeton University Press, 1992) 186.

succession five of my siblings. My relationship with my father broke down. I took some time out, travelling north from Copenhagen to the coast, and thought about the kind of person I wanted to be. While staying in the charming seaside village of Gilleleje in August 1835, I wrote in my diary: 'What I really need is to get clear about what I must do, not what I must know… the crucial thing is to find a truth which is truth for me, to find the idea for which I am willing to live and die.'[2]

By the way, I know what it means to work from home; in fact, I worked from home all of my adult life. In my case however, it was not from compulsion, but from convenience. I inherited enough money from my father to enable me to live as a writer without having to hold down a day job, and I was able to publish all my books at my own expense. Just as well, because most of my books were financial flops. My contemporaries simply weren't ready for me: I went against the current and was too far ahead of my time. As I once noted in my diary, 'People understand me so little that they do not even understand my laments over their not understanding me'.[3]

But in case you think I got off lightly by having had the leisure to work from home, let me add that for several years I was obliged to socially distance myself, even though there was no pandemic raging at the time. After I got into a dispute with *The Corsair*, a satirical newspaper, the paper began to make fun of me with cruel cartoons and caricatures. I could no longer walk around Copenhagen because passers-by ridiculed me, and young boys hurled stones in my direction.

Passion

They made fun of me because I stood for something rather than falling for everything. I was a man of passion. I want to ask you – where has your passion gone? To find your passion you must find yourself. And to find yourself, you need silence. That's why in my book *For Self-Examination* I wrote: 'in observing the present state

2   Søren Kierkegaard, *Søren Kierkegaard's Journals and Papers*, edited and translated by Howard and Edna Hong (Bloomington: Indiana University Press, 1968), Volume 5, Entry Number 5100.
3   Ibid., 5119.

of the world and life in general, from a Christian point of view one has to say: it is a disease. And if I were a physician and someone asked me, "What do you think should be done?" I would answer, "the first thing ... the very first thing that must be done is: create silence, bring about silence. God's Word cannot be heard, and if in order to be heard in the hullabaloo it must be shouted deafeningly with noisy instruments, then it is not God's Word; create silence!"[4] This existential crisis is your opportunity to turn your attention inwards, to dig deeper than the surface layer of chatter and gossip, to find the silence that helps you to find yourself.

Your English word 'passion' comes from the Latin word for suffering. Keep in mind that passion entails a struggle: it's about the struggle of swimming against the tide by believing something that others dismiss as stupidity. If you decide not to swim against the tide, you might as well resign yourself right now to being a corpse, because corpses always follow the flow!

The Bible is full of passion. But most of you Christians today don't want to understand the Bible, because you know very well that the moment you understand it, you will be obliged to put it into practice. And so you have invented biblical scholarship to defend yourselves against the Bible, to ensure that you can continue to be respectable Christians without the Bible coming too close. 'I open the New Testament and read: "If you want to be perfect, go, sell all your goods and give to the poor, and come, follow me" (Mt 19:21). Good God, if we were to actually do this, all the capitalists, the office holders and the entrepreneurs, the whole society in fact, would be almost beggars! We would be sunk if it were not for Christian scholarship! Praise be to everyone who works to consolidate the reputation of Christian scholarship, which helps to restrain the New Testament, this confounded book which would one, two, three, run us all down if it got loose (that is, if Christian scholarship did not restrain it).'[5]

---

4   Søren Kierkegaard, *For Self-Examination*, edited and translated by Howard and Edna Hong (Princeton: Princeton University Press, 1990), 47.
5   Søren Kierkegaard in *Provocations: Spiritual Writings of Kierkegaard*, compiled and edited by Charles E. Moore (New York: Plough, 2007) 201-202.

If you don't profit from this pandemic to revive the passion of your faith, you'll sink even further into a bog of mediocrity. The greatest danger to Christianity doesn't come from atheists or secularists or heretics. No, the worst danger trickles out from the kind of orthodoxy that is nothing but honeyed drivel, mediocrity with a dash of sugar, always polite, always cordial, but so inoffensive that it might as well not exist.

Have you really lived your own life? Or are you just following the crowd? Whose opinions come out of your mouth? Are they really your own or are they second-hand truths that you have unthinkingly absorbed? This COVID-19 crisis is your chance to ascend above the green meadow gregariousness of bovine mediocrity!

Suffering and anxiety
But first you must suffer. Yes, you heard me right – suffer. Let me be clear, clearer than I used to be during my own lifetime. First, suffering without Christ is just a waste of time. Second, when I speak about suffering, I don't mean physical pain, but the suffering of the mind and of the spirit. Without a spirit, there is no suffering, only pain. True suffering is to leave your ego aside, because the only way to relate to the Absolute is absolutely. It's not enough to accept just one side of Christianity by seeking out a life of pleasure, and then paint up this lying style of life as pure Christianity. How can you imitate Christ if your only quest is for comfort and ease?

If your religion remains at the level of mediocrity, you will be too afraid to meet Christ on the way of the Cross. Mediocrity is a disease that stops you lifting yourself up from self-centred concerns. But if you respond promptly and courageously to Christ's call to follow him, you'll discover, as I did, that the way is strewn with unsuspected graces, turning your suffering into joy.

It sounds cruel, but I hope this pandemic is already making you suffer, because you will only begin to wake up to the truth through suffering. Remember the prodigal son? It was only when he started suffering that he decided to return to his father. People can perform extraordinary feats and yet be devoid of any understanding of themselves. But suffering directs our gaze within. If it succeeds, that is the start of real learning, the learning that comes from the rough and tumble school of life. Do you imagine that you can arrive easily at the truth? That you can dream your way to it? No, you must be tested, you must fight the good fight, and suffer if you are to reach the truth. It is sheer fantasy to imagine that there is a pain-free short-cut to what is most important in life.

My own father Michael reared me in a severe way. When he disciplined me as a child, explaining why the things I did were wrong, often at the time I didn't understand the point he was making. It was only much later that I saw the method in his madness. In a similar way, when God disciplines you now, you may not grasp the purpose immediately. But trust him, because sooner or later this purpose will be revealed.

I'd recommend that you learn not to resist the suffering of anxiety. Be prepared to walk through the valley of anxiety, without fearing evil and without looking nervously behind your back every other minute. If you grasp the opportunity that lies hidden in the anxiety of this pandemic, you may just find your way to a more authentic life.

Don't prematurely judge anxiety as something merely negative. The truth is that anxiety is the reverse side of something essentially positive – the fact that you are human. To be human is to have possibilities, and whenever you have possibilities, you have anxiety as well. You have the possibility of becoming a real grown-up, but in order to do so, you must leave aside childish ways – and dropping childish ways causes anxiety. You have the possibility of becoming your true self, but in order to do so, you must leave aside the false self, and removing the false self from the driving seat causes anxiety. Although deep down you know that this immature self imprisons you, the prison has become so comfortable that you are reluctant to escape. The patterns of your past are thoroughly ingrained; no wonder you feel anxiety at the prospect of choosing to be a little grain of wheat that falls into the ground and dies.

The suffering of anxiety is actually a proof of your nobility. Even though it is demanding to live with the suffering of anxiety, it nevertheless shows that you are more than a mere beast, that you have a spiritual nature. In my carefree student days, I tried to distract myself from the spiritual dimension of life. I raced after superficialities, yet I couldn't help feeling the gnawing emptiness inside. I remember going to a party. It seemed so enjoyable, but when I returned home, I found myself penning this harrowing sentence: 'I have just returned from a party of which I was the life and soul; wit poured from my lips, everyone laughed and admired me – but I went away – and the dash should be as long as the earth's orbit – and wanted to shoot myself.'[6] It's so tempting – and so easy – to lose sight of your true dignity, and to smother the genuine hungers of your life. I wrote something to that effect in my book *The Sickness unto Death*: 'the greatest hazard of all, losing the self, can occur very quietly in the world, as if it were nothing at all. No other loss can occur so quietly; any other loss – an arm, a leg, five dollars, a wife, etc. – is sure to be noticed.'[7]

I was saved from the silent danger of losing my soul through the vocal love of a woman, Regine Olsen. We loved each other deeply. But my love for her awakened me to an even greater love, the love of God. Breaking my engagement with her caused huge anxiety for me – and immense suffering for Regine. Yet it was actually my way of becoming engaged to God. My eccentricity didn't disappear as a result, but I thank God that this marvellous woman helped my soul escape from prison so that I learned to channel my passion for writing and language into God's service.

So I say to you: anxiety isn't a door that closes your way to freedom; rather, it's a window opening up a huge world of possibilities. The greatest possibility to which anxiety can open up your life is – God. So instead of running in the opposite direction when you see anxiety coming, take your anxiety and bring it before God, trusting that God

6   Søren Kierkegaard, *The Soul of Kierkegaard: Selections from his Journals*, edited and with an introduction by Alexander Dru (Mineola, NY: Dover Publications, 2003) 50–51.
7   Søren Kierkegaard, *The Sickness Unto Death*, edited and translated by Howard and Edna Hong, with introduction and notes (Princeton: Princeton University Press, 1980) 32–33.

is trustworthy. You need to learn how to use your anxiety in the best way possible, by seeing it as an invitation to turn to God in a spirit of immense confidence. So don't allow anxiety to degenerate into panic; instead, make it rise into prayer.

A passionate appeal

What does it mean to rise into prayer instead of descending into panic? The following story of mine throws light on this issue, because it shows that our destiny is to take to the sky rather than to remain grounded. And it also shows that taking our destiny seriously is a costly affair, though not nearly as costly as refusing to fly.

'Try to imagine for a moment that geese could talk – that they had so arranged things that they too had their divine worship and their church-going. Every Sunday they would meet together, and a gander would preach. The sermon was essentially the same each time – it told of the glorious destiny of geese, of the noble end for which their maker had created them – and every time his name was mentioned all the geese curtsied and all the ganders bowed their heads. They were to use their wings to fly away to the distant pastures to which they really belonged; for they were only pilgrims on this earth. The same thing happened each Sunday. Thereupon the meeting broke up and they all waddled home, only to meet again next Sunday for divine worship and waddle off home again – but that was as far as they ever got. They throve and grew fat, plump and delicious – and at Michaelmas they were eaten – and that was as far as they ever got. It never came to anything. For while their conversation on Sundays was high-sounding, on Mondays they would tell each other what had happened to the goose who had taken the end set before them quite seriously, and in spite of many tribulations had tried to use the wings its creator had bestowed upon it... Among the geese were several who looked ill and wan, and all the other geese said – there, you see what comes of taking flying seriously. It is all because they go about meditating on flying that they get thin and wan and are not blessed by the grace of God as we are; for that is why we grow fat, plump and delicious...

'So it is with our Christian worship services. We, too, have wings, we have imagination, intended to help us actually rise aloft. But we play, allow our imagination to amuse itself in an hour of Sunday daydreaming. In reality, however, we stay right where we are – and on Monday regard it as a proof that God's grace gets us plump, fat, delicate. That is, we accumulate money, get to be a somebody in the world, beget children, become successful, and so forth. And those who actually get involved with God and who therefore suffer and have torments, troubles, and grief, of these we say: Here is proof that they do not have the grace of God.'[8]

One reason I chose geese as the focus of that moral tale was because of my lifelong passion for nature, a passion to which most scholars give little or no attention. But just leaf (yes, this choice of verb is deliberate!) through my voluminous journals and you'll discover how deeply I loved God's creation. Many of you had the opportunity during the lockdowns to get in touch with nature in a new way: for instance, by being able to hear clearly for the first time an amazing variety of birdsong. My fear is that you will learn little from this newfound connection with nature. And if you don't learn from the pandemic, how will you be ready to make the changes necessary to tackle the environmental crisis?

Read the following parable, and then I'll explain how it can be seen as a passionate appeal to take radical action to protect our planet. This parable appears in *Either / Or*, the only book of mine that sold reasonably well during my lifetime: 'In a theatre, it happened that a fire started offstage. The clown came out to tell the audience. They thought it was a joke and applauded. He told them again, and they became still more hilarious. This is the way, I believe, that the world will be destroyed – amidst the universal hilarity of wits and wags who think it is all a joke.'[9]

The recent pandemic has been likened to a dress rehearsal for

8   Søren Kierkegaard, *Journals*, edited and translated by Alexander Dru (New York: Harper Torchbooks, 1959) 252–53.
9   Søren Kierkegaard, *Either/Or, Part I*, edited and translated by Howard and Edna Hong, with introduction and notes (Princeton: Princeton University Press, 1987) 30.

the ultimate existential threat that is climate change. I say ultimate because it's a much greater threat and one that could lead to the extinction of *homo sapiens*, as it has done and continues to do for so many other species.

Both threats have much in common, but they differ in two significant respects.

Firstly, you knew there was a risk of a massive viral outbreak, yet when it came, it arrived with little or no warning. Not so with climate change! There are ample warnings that it's real and that it's unfolding.

Secondly, unlike the pandemic, there is no vaccine for climate change tipping points, such as the shutting down of the Gulf Stream due to an increased influx of freshwater to the North Atlantic; the changes they bring to countries such as Denmark and Ireland will be abrupt and irreversible.

Those countries that heed the science and data, are responding best to the pandemic. Who is heeding the scientific evidence that climate change is adverse, global, and largely driven by human beings?

I hope by the time that you, the audience, eventually wake up and listen to the call of the clown, there'll still be time to mitigate its threat to life and to this planet.

Questions for Reflection and Discussion

1. If we reflect on our own lives, have we lost our passion for the important things?
2. In order to find ourselves, are we able to make time for silence?
3. Are we really living our own lives, or are we just following the crowd?
4. In our own situation, can we view anxiety positively – not as a door that closes our way to freedom, but rather as a window opening up a huge world of possibilities?

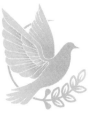

Do Not Be Afraid
to Give Your Time to Christ

Neil Xavier O'Donoghue

'*Who* said Mass?' reads the post displayed in 2020 on the *Irish Mammy Sayings* wall in Dublin Airport. Going to Mass on Sunday used to be considered as a mark of Irishness, but in recent years the number of Catholics attending Sunday Mass in Ireland has diminished. Before the COVID-19 lockdowns, Sunday Mass attendance had fallen to well under 50%, with some reporting an attendance of less than 20% in Dublin. Most people would agree that these numbers are not likely to go up in the near future.[1]

I remember as a child in the Seventies being told that I was expected to be physically present in church from the Gospel until when the priest received Communion. I also remember how some men who were at the back of the church would leave the moment that the priest received Communion. Yet Mass attendance was ubiquitous in the Ireland of my childhood. When John Paul II celebrated Mass in Dublin's Phoenix Park during his 1979 visit he was to comment

---

1 From a historical perspective it is untrue to state that Mass attendance numbers were always high in Ireland. In fact, they have fluctuated over the centuries, with some historians proposing very low attendance prior to the Great Irish Famine. Miller has produced evidence for 1834 which shows that while some parts of Ireland had very high Mass attendance, many places, particularly in the West of Ireland, had an average Sunday Mass attendance of only 30%. David W. Miller, 'Mass attendance in Ireland in 1834', in Stewart J. Brown and David W. Miller, eds., *Piety and Power in Ireland, 1760–1960: Essays in Honour of Emmet Larkin* (Notre Dame, IN: University of Notre Dame Press, 2000), 158–179.

that 'on Sunday mornings in Ireland, no one seeing the great crowds making their way to and from Mass could have any doubt about Ireland's devotion to the Mass'. Nowadays 'great crowds' attending Mass are a rare occurrence – associated with the earliest Mass on Christmas Eve or the odd funeral.

In March 2020, as the world seemed to close down overnight, Ireland embarked on a severe lockdown to combat transmission of the virus. As part of this national effort the Catholic Church cancelled all public Masses and, in many places, the churches were even locked. Public Masses would not resume until the very end of June 2020, just to be stopped again months later. At the height of the pandemic only severely restricted funeral Masses with a minimum of people were allowed. Many priests streamed their private Masses on Zoom or Facebook Live, and RTÉ's daily Mass was a remarkable success with very high viewing numbers. While many people availed of these, and others marked Sunday with private devotions, my impression is that a high percentage of people who had regularly attended Mass every week or every few weeks, didn't bother availing of any of these options and simply lived Sunday as any other day.

Many have commented on the harm that loneliness, fear and depression associated with the lockdown did to so many people. On the practical level, some have underlined the economic challenge that many parishes and religious institutions face in the wake of losing their main source of revenue. Indeed, it is likely that the COVID experience has accelerated the process of secularisation in Ireland and Mass attendance numbers won't return to the 2019 levels any time soon. But in this chapter, I propose that the COVID crisis has revealed how the very institution of Sunday is in crisis in Irish Catholicism and I offer some initial reflections on how we can begin to reappreciate its importance.

While there are many people of a deep faith in Ireland, the uncomfortable truth is that for many Catholics, the half hour or so they spent in church on a Sunday morning is often the full extent of the practice of the faith. Obviously, there is much more to being a Christian than formal religious practice, but we must avoid the extreme of equating Christianity with civic-mindedness or being a good neighbour. The local GAA clubs did some fantastic work helping the elderly and house-bound during the lockdowns. But I think it would be an exaggeration to claim that this great work was undertaken as a fruit of the members' Christian faith. If many baptised Catholics do not nourish their spiritual lives for months on end, is it an exaggeration to say that they no longer practise their faith, no matter how nice they are?

Sundays in Christian tradition

Since the earliest days of Christianity, Sunday has had a special role in Christian identity. Indeed, Christians could be said to be those who observe the Lord's Day. The Christian Sunday is related to the Old Testament institution of the Sabbath. The first account of creation in Genesis tells us that God 'rested on the seventh day from all the work that he had done. So God blessed the seventh day and hallowed it, because on it God rested from all the work that he had done in creation' (Gen 2:2–3).

As God had rested on the Seventh Day, unsurprisingly the People of Israel were also called to rest as an *imitatio Dei*, or imitation of God. Throughout the Old Testament period the Sabbath was to develop and by the time of Jesus it had come to symbolise what it meant to be a Jew. Together with the Temple, the Sabbath became one of the central institutions of the Old Testament and to this day marks the identity of Israel. [2]

But gradually the Sabbath rest had become absolute. Paradoxically the rest was to become a burden. The Book of Exodus prescribes the death penalty for working on the Sabbath: 'Six days shall work be done, but on the seventh day you shall have a holy Sabbath of solemn rest to the Lord; whoever does any work on it shall be put to death' (Ex 35:2, see Num 15:35). During the Maccabean Revolt some of

---

2   For a beautiful reflection on the role of the Sabbath in recent Judaism, see Abraham Joshua Heschel, *The Sabbath: Its Meaning for Modern Man* (New York: Farrar, Straus and Giroux, 1951).

the Jewish rebels preferred to let themselves be slaughtered by the pagans rather than break the Sabbath law to protect themselves in self-defence (see 1 Macc 2:29–41).

In the New Testament, Jesus was to oppose a wooden observance of the Sabbath (Mk 3:1–6). He was to rescue humanity from an oppressive Sabbath rest. Indeed, in contrast to the burdensome Sabbath, he proclaimed, 'Come to me, all you that are weary and are carrying heavy burdens, and I will give you rest. Take my yoke upon you and learn from me; for I am gentle and humble in heart, and you will find rest for your souls. For my yoke is easy, and my burden is light' (Mt 11:28–30). He even went so far as to proclaim, 'the Sabbath was made for humankind, and not humankind for the Sabbath' (Mk 2:27). This reinvention of the Sabbath was one of the reasons behind Jesus' conflict with the religious authorities, and perhaps even one of the reasons that Jesus was condemned to death (Jn 5:18).

But in the New Testament, the Sabbath is fulfilled not by the Christian Sunday but in Jesus Christ himself (Col 2:16–17). In this sense, Sunday is a totally new reality. In the earliest Church, Christians did not rest on a Sabbath-like Sunday, but they celebrated the Christ event. It was the first day, the day of the resurrection. In the Roman world where the first Christians lived, Sunday was not a day off and, even if they had so desired, most Christians simply could not refrain from work.

While the New Testament doesn't give too many details about Sunday, it does seem that it was the specific day that Christians gathered together for worship (see Acts 20:6–11, 1 Cor 16:1–2). In the beginning of the Book of Revelation, John tells us that he received his vision on the 'Lord's Day' (Rev 1:10). Clearly this day was a very special day for the first Christians. Joseph Ratzinger comments on how 'Sunday, the first day of the week (also regarded as the first day of creation and now marking the new creation) is the real inner locus of the Eucharist as a Christian form. Sunday and Eucharist belong together right from the beginning; the day of the

Resurrection is the matrix of the Eucharist'. [3]

The *Didache*, the earliest Christian catechetical manual dating from the end of the first century, already takes it for granted that Christians gather together to celebrate the Eucharist on Sunday: 'On the Lord's own day gather together and break bread and give thanks, having first confessed your sins so that your sacrifice may be pure'. [4] St Justin Martyr, writing his famous account of the Christian Eucharist around the year 155, also tells us that the Christians gathered for the Eucharist on Sunday mornings. [5] Gathering together to celebrate the Lord's Day was to become a hallmark of Christianity. When Pliny the Younger was giving an account of the Christians to the Emperor Trajan early in the second century, he mentioned that they gathered on a specific day. [6]

When the Roman State was persecuting Christians, one tactic they used to catch the Christians red-handed was to see who gathered together secretly on a Sunday morning. In a famous example during the persecution of Diocletian in Abitinae, North Africa, in the year 304 a large group of Christians were arrested as they gathered to celebrate Mass. During their trial, a Christian named Emeritus, the soon to be martyred owner of the house where the Eucharist was celebrated, was asked why he allowed this illegal gathering in his property. His answer captures the experience of Sunday in the early Church. He told the proconsul that he couldn't stop the celebration in his house for '*sine dominico non possumus* – without the Day of the Lord, we cannot exist'. [7]

Yet over the centuries this clear vision of Sunday as the day of the Resurrection of Christ was gradually lost. Initially this may have

3   Joseph Ratzinger, *The Feast of Faith: Approaches to a Theology of the Liturgy*, trans. Graham Harrison (San Francisco: Ignatius Press, 1986), 45.
4   *Didache* 14 in Michael William Holmes, *The Apostolic Fathers: Greek Texts and English Translations*, Updated ed. (Grand Rapids, MI: Baker Books, 1999), 267.
5   St Justin, *Apology* 1, 65–67; the text is conveniently quoted in the *Catechism of the Catholic Church*, 1355.
6   Robert Louis Wilken, *The Christians as the Romans Saw Them* (New Haven, CT: Yale University Press, 2003), 19.
7   Quoted in Joseph Cardinal Ratzinger, *A New Song for the Lord: Faith in Christ and Liturgy Today* (New York: Crossroad, 1996), 60.

been an unintended consequence of the Emperor Constantine's law of 321 when he prohibited public work on Sundays, partly as a concession to the newly legalised Christians. Elements of the Old Testament Sabbath were adopted by Christians, and for most Christians, Sunday became their Sabbath. Many of the sometimes-onerous Old Testament laws on Sabbath observance were applied to the Christian Sunday. This was particularly evident in the Church in pre-Norman Ireland where there was a firm insistence on abstaining from any work or chore on Sunday. [8] This strong emphasis on Sunday as a day of rest, with strict regulations governing behaviour was to become a central part of the spirituality of some Protestant Churches, where to this day members of some denominations are expected to spend most of Sunday in church. But while the Catholic Church has appropriated the idea of Sunday as a day of rest, it has always stressed the importance of attending the Eucharist, eventually defining Sunday Mass attendance as a precept of the Church. [9] Indeed, for much of the history of the Church the meaning of Sunday can be well summarised in the words of the famous 1951 *Maynooth Catechism*: 'the Church commands us to keep holy the Lord's day by assisting at Mass and abstaining from servile work'.

A renewal of Sunday
The Second Vatican Council speaks about Sunday in the *Constitution on the Liturgy*, where number 106 states that:

> By a tradition handed down from the apostles which took its origin from the very day of Christ's resurrection, the Church celebrates the paschal mystery every eighth day; with good reason this, then, bears the name of the Lord's day or Sunday. For on this day Christ's faithful are bound to

---

8 For a selection of texts see Neil Xavier O'Donoghue, *The Eucharist in Pre-Norman Ireland* (Notre Dame, IN: University of Notre Dame Press, 2011), 130–133.

9 A general history of magisterial statements on Sunday is provided in Shawn Madigan, 'Sunday' in Joseph A. Komonchak, Mary Collins, and Dermot A. Lane, eds., *The New Dictionary of Theology* (Collegeville, MN: Liturgical Press, 2000), 992–995.

come together into one place so that, by hearing the word of God and taking part in the Eucharist, they may call to mind the passion, the resurrection and the glorification of the Lord Jesus, and may thank God who "has begotten them again, through the resurrection of Jesus Christ from the dead, unto a living hope". Hence the Lord's day is the original feast day, and it should be proposed to the piety of the faithful and taught to them so that it may become in fact a day of joy and of freedom from work. [10]

This renewed emphasis on Sunday was seen in the *Roman Calendar* and the *Roman Missal* as revised under Pope Paul VI. However, on an official level, attendance at Mass was still promoted as a precept of the Church. The *Catechism of the Catholic Church* still states that the first Church precept is that 'You shall attend Mass on Sundays and on holy days of obligation and rest from servile labour' (CCC, 2042); this forms part of 'the very necessary minimum" of what it means to be considered a Catholic in good standing. The 1983 *Code of Canon Law* still uses the word 'obligation' for attendance at Mass (CIC, 1247).

While on a juridical level this is true, I propose that we need to go further. The Catholic faith cannot be reduced to an obligation to go to Mass. While attendance at Mass is a very important element of what Christian tradition tells us about what Sunday is, it is only one part of the equation. Indeed, Eastern Catholics can fulfil their 'Sunday Obligation' by participating in the Liturgy of the Hours in their local church instead of going to Mass (see *The Code of Canons of the Eastern Churches*, 881). Prior to Vatican II, traditional devotions, such as Benediction and Novenas were common and almost as well attended as Mass itself. [11]

However after the Council, there was a tendency to leave these

10   See the Vatican website: www.vatican.va/archive/hist_councils/ii_vatican_council/documents/vat-ii_const_19631204_sacrosanctum-concilium_en.html.

11   For a recollection of parish life in Ireland in the 1950s see Eamon Duffy, *Faith of our Fathers: Reflections on Catholic Tradition* (London: Continuum, 2004), 20–28.

devotions and celebrate Mass on every religious occasion. It is true that the Mass is the 'source and summit of the Christian life' (*Lumen Gentium,* 11), but it is not the entirety of the Church's spiritual treasury. An overreliance on the Mass over the last fifty years has led to an unhealthy clericalism, where many Catholics feel that the only thing that counts is going to Mass. All too often priests and other Catholic leaders have stressed Sunday Mass attendance as the necessary minimum, and all too often this has been understood by those being preached to as being the only thing necessary. This has led to an almost magical, one-dimensional social Catholicism that has been shorn of its great spiritual tradition and Catholics who think their Christianity depends on being physically present in the church for half an hour on a Sunday morning. This is a far cry from the discipleship that Christ preached, inviting us to be transformed day by day into his own likeness.

The lockdown was a time when Catholics were unable to attend Mass. I would propose that many people were spiritually orphaned in this time and their faith lives suffered greatly. There is a true crisis of faith in the Church today. All too many Catholics have no real relationship with the Word of God. While they might listen to the readings and the homily when they are in church, they do not read the Bible (or maybe even own one). Even fewer people own a copy of the *Divine Office* or are even aware of its existence. Some apps such as Universalis or iBreviary are popular enough, but those who use them only make up a drop in the ocean of the world's Catholics. Likewise, monthly publications such as *Magnificat* or *Give us This Day* have a simplified version of the Liturgy of the Hours, but these are only purchased by the most devout. Some families still pray a family rosary, but for most the rosary is a strange relic of a Catholic past. Many of the young see it simply as a piece of Catholic jewellery or a talisman and couldn't pray on its beads if their life depended on it.

While there are many valid ways to pray and to nourish our relationship with God, all of us need to select a few of these options and regularly use them as the basis of our spiritual life. The Mass may be the 'source and summit' of the spiritual life, but it cannot be the sum total of that spiritual life. Our Lord has said to us that 'where two or three are gathered in my name, I am there among them' (Mt 18:20). But there was no widespread evidence of people gathering in twos and threes to pray together while the churches were closed. Irish Catholics simply seem to be unaware of this promise of Christ. Most practicing Catholics tend to simply 'get Mass'. There is all too little awareness that a community is involved in the celebration of Mass. Pope John Paul II warned that 'the anonymity of the city cannot be allowed to enter our Eucharistic communities'. [12] Once upon a time, at least in a village or small town, everyone knew everyone, and a parish would notice if someone missed Mass. Nowadays in many Irish parishes, people can go to Mass without any interaction with another person. At most there is a handshake at the sign of peace, but people are anonymous and usually wouldn't be missed if they didn't come.

Another aspect of the crisis is that even prior to the COVID-19 shutdown, Sunday had lost a lot of its meaning. Sunday needs to be special for Christians. When Ireland was a poorer country, the wearing of better clothes on Sunday, your 'Sunday best', helped mark the day as special. Also the Sunday dinner, which was of a better quality than weekdays, helped give a festive touch to the day. Today many of us can eat what we want when we want, but in our abundance, we have lost the experience of Sunday as a feast.

While many people still have a Monday to Friday working week, there is now nothing unusual in having shops and an increasing number of businesses open on Sundays. We feel that workers can take their weekend at another time in the week, and certain jobs will offer better pay for working on Sunday. But as Christians, we ought to examine our conscience about whether we ourselves patronise businesses unnecessarily on a Sunday. It isn't a matter of picketing the local supermarket or petrol station to protest against Sunday-trading, but deciding about the type of life we ourselves

---

12 Address of John Paul II to the Bishops of Ontario (Canada) on Their *Ad Limina* Visit, 4 May 1999, available at w2.vatican.va/content/john–paul–ii/en/speeches/1999/may/documents/ hf_jp–ii_spe_19990504_ad–limina–canada–ontario.html.

live and the values we espouse as Christians.

It would also be good for us to think about how we live Sunday in our own homes. Many of us live hectic lives and, even if we don't go to our place of employment on a Sunday, it is perhaps the day when we work the most, catching up on our cleaning and laundry, as well as running all of our errands. Sunday can also be a day of special solidarity with the poor and the sick. It can be a good day to visit those who need company and also an opportunity to invite people to our own homes for a meal. Loneliness is an epidemic in modern society and Christian families are called to help those who are by themselves, knowing that when we entertain the less fortunate, we often welcome angels into our homes (see Heb 13:2).

When public Masses were celebrated under the social distancing rules after the easing of the lockdowns, some churches didn't have the capacity to fit everyone who wanted to attend Sunday Mass. This situation led to people being turned away from the church doors in many parishes. In the circumstances, this was understandable and unavoidable. In response some people decided to go to Mass on a weekday instead of Sunday. While this might work as a short-term solution, in the long term we cannot simply say that Sunday has been replaced with everyone attending Mass as a private act of devotion on whatever day of the week fits better into their social calendar. We are not saved by ourselves, but as members of a community that is the Church of Christ!

Perhaps we can better appreciate the importance of Sunday from a 2018 catechesis that Pope Francis gave on the Third Commandment. He stressed the vital role of rest for a healthy human life. This is a challenge because 'true rest is not simple, because there is false rest and true rest'. Undoubtedly, there is a universal desire for rest and, as Pope Francis explains, 'today's society thirsts for amusement and holidays ... The prevailing concept of *life* today does not have its centre of gravity in activity and commitment, but in *escapism*. Earning money to have fun, to satisfy oneself'. This leads us to the paradoxical situation whereby 'people have never rested as much as today, yet they have never experienced as much emptiness as today!'

The basic problem is that in spite of all that the modern world has to offer, these things 'do not give [us] fullness of heart, indeed: they do not give [us] rest'. The Pope proposes that on Sunday we are invited to experience 'true' rest, which 'is the moment of contemplation, it is the moment of praise, not that of escapism'. Sunday 'is the time to look at reality and say: how beautiful life is! Contrary to rest as an escape from reality, the Decalogue proposes rest as the *blessing of reality*'. The Holy Father continues relating the element of rest to the celebration of the Eucharist. 'For us Christians,' he says, 'the centre of the Lord's day, Sunday, is the Eucharist, which means "thanksgiving". It is the day to say to God: thank you Lord for life, for your mercy, for all your gifts. Sunday is not the day to forget the other days but to remember them, bless them and make peace with life.' [13]

If our goal is simply to go back to where we were in February 2020, before the COVID-19 lockdown, then the Church in Ireland will surely die. We must endeavour to become a people in passionate love with Christ and transformed by his resurrection, who can live the Lord's Day as the centre of their week and their being.

Questions for Reflection and Discussion

1. How do I live Sunday? To what degree is it a special day or is it, at best, a day of religious obligation?
2. How can we as a parish encourage a deeper appreciation of the Bible and the Liturgy of the Hours and other forms of personal prayer?
3. How do we help make society less busy on Sundays?
4. Do I use Sunday as a day to do good for others? Is it a self-centred day which I use for chores or self-satisfaction? Do I help others to rest on Sunday, or does my lifestyle make it harder for others to properly live this day?

---

13 See Pope Francis' General Audience on Wednesday, 5 September 2018 available at http://www.vatican.va/content/francesco/en/audiences/2018/documents/papa-francesco_20180905_udienza-generale.html.

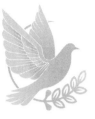

COVID-19 and the
Spiritual Lives of Children

John-Paul Sheridan

The pandemic has been a weighty burden on children in so many different ways, including their religious education and catechesis. In the majority of schools / parishes the religious education programme was halted on lockdown, and parents 'stepped up to the plate' when it came to schoolwork in some of the primary school subjects. Teachers valiantly gave parents schoolwork for their children, including work from the *Grow in Love* programme.

Furthermore, sacramental preparation was halted, and the annual celebrations of the Sacraments of First Holy Communion, First Reconciliation and Confirmation were generally put on hold, in some cases, more than once. This was difficult for children and their families, despite assurances from parishes that celebrations were deferred and not postponed. Parishes became creative during the lockdown in attempting to facilitate the child's 'special day'. However, while the domestic Church in lockdown might not have access to sacraments, it does still have moments in which the sacramentality of life and family can make real and present the person of Jesus Christ.

Writers on the spirituality of the child have something to offer in relation to the child in the COVID-19 pandemic and their overall spiritual development, so that even if the religious education programme is set aside, there are still opportunities to nurture the spiritual lives of children. Normally I will offer students preparing to teach in primary schools some of the writing on children's spirituality as a way to best prepare them for working with children in their future classrooms. The purpose is to help them understand that a child is not just an undeveloped adult, and that the spiritual lives of children are just as worthy of note as the spiritual lives of adults. In fact, it is worth considering these young spiritual lives as a reminder to ourselves of what we might have lost as we grow older.

This chapter focuses on children's spiritual lives and how they might be nourished and strengthened even in a time of crisis and uncertainty. I will begin with a few remarks regarding the spiritual life of children from some of the current contributions to the field. I will then offer some thoughts on learning and celebrating in the domestic church, especially with children who had been preparing for the celebration of sacraments. I will consider the way parents and families can accompany children in their spiritual journey, even in a lockdown.

The spiritual life of the child

> At night, a lot, I'll be looking out the window, and it's real quiet, and you can sit and wonder if there are people like you up on other planets or stars; and you can wonder whether there is a God watching you – or maybe there are several gods, or lots of them, or angels, I don't know, but I think about it, and how it's not fair ... that you and I are healthy, and others, your brother aren't.

This is part of an interview that the psychologist Robert Coles undertook with a twelve-year-old boy called Norman.[1] The quotation here is a strong example of many of the aspects of children's spirituality which are important for teachers and parents to understand.

---

1   Robert Coles, *The Spiritual Life of Children* (Boston, MA: Houghton Mifflin, 1990) 298. Cited in Heather Nicole Ingersoll, 'Making Room: A Place for Children's Spirituality in the Christian Church,' *International Journal of Children's Spirituality* 19:3–4 (2014) 164-178, here 164.

Norman is trying to understand why his brother is sick and he is not. Rather than asking the question directly, he begins a questing of sorts and starts far out in the universe. As he gradually focuses in, he is questioning a great deal and trying, within the limitations of the twelve-year-old intellect to comprehend God, angels and everything else. I use the word limitations, but that is not to say that Norman is limited in the ability his imagination has to think and to try and create connections between what seems to be the fundamental issue for him and his thoughts on the meaning of life. Brendan Hyde describes children's spirituality in four specific characteristics: felt sense, integrating awareness, weaving threads of meaning and spiritual questing.[2] These characteristics sum up Norman's interview with Coles. We can see that his questioning is both genuine and heartfelt. In attempting to come to a satisfactory understanding of why his brother is sick and he is not, Norman begins far out in the universe and eventually funnels down to the heart of his question.

Machteld Reynaert defines children's spirituality as the 'capacity children initially possess to search for meaning in their lives'.[3] This is embedded in the everyday life of the child and has influence over the life of the child and shapes the child's way of being. Rebecca Nye offers this: 'a very simple definition of children's spirituality might be: God's way of being with children and children's ways of being with God'.[4] She goes on to suggest that children's spirituality begins with God and not with adults, as God is their creator. From this point of departure, she moves on to some specific features, defining it as an 'initially natural capacity for awareness of the sacred quality of life experiences'.[5]

Experiences are key in a child's attempts to understand the

---

2   Brendan Hyde, 'The Identification of Four Characteristics of Children's Spirituality in Australian Catholic Primary Schools,' *International Journal of Children's Spirituality* 13:2 (2008) 117–127, here 120.
3   Machteld Reynaert, 'Pastoral Power in Nurturing the Spiritual Life of the Child,' *International Journal of Children's Spirituality* 19:3–4 (2014) 179–186, here 179.
4   Rebecca Nye, *Children's Spirituality, What It Is and Why It Matters* (London: Church House Publishing, 2009), 5.
5   Ibid., 6.

world, even experiences sadly lacking in a 'sacred' quality. The work of the Turkish artist Erkan Özgen comes to mind. Titled *Wonderland* (2016)[6], this short film / art installation shows a young boy, Muhammed, describing the war in Syria, capturing the intense horror the boy has witnessed. 'Muhammed's gestures start from the initial demonstrations against the regime, then the war, which we know has multiple layers and actors that led to massive destruction and migration in Syria'.[7] The boy is deaf and mute and while unfamiliar with the conventions of International Sign Language, he can manage to describe vividly in movements that are almost ballet-like. One can only begin to imagine how a child can process what he has witnessed. Every day, children look at the world around and seek to make connection between their experience and some of the spiritual and existential questions that come across their radar from time to time. This rich web of experience is one that educators and parents can draw on when helping the child make sense of their spiritual identity.

Tony Eaude (echoing Linda Hogg and Berry Mayall[8]) believes that schools 'too often do not draw on the children's "funds of knowledge" – what they bring from experience outside school – and that to do so is especially motivating for those disengaged from school learning'.[9] Children love to ask questions; indeed, anyone who has ever been in the company of a child will be familiar with their ability to question. While this might seem to be annoying or tedious at times, it is both the questioning imagination of the child and their ease and comfort with the adult which facilitates this dialogue. As well as seeing this as a dialogue, it is also useful to see it in terms of a journey.

6   This video can be found on YouTube simply through a search for the title and artist's name.
7   Cihad Caner, 'Is it possible to represent war without violent images?', *Daily Sabah*, 8/04/19
8   Linda Hogg, 'Funds of Knowledge: An Investigation of Coherence within the Literature'. *Teaching and Teacher Education* 27 (2011) 666–677; Berry Mayall, 'Children's Lives Outside School and Their Educational Impact', *The Cambridge Primary Review Research Surveys*, edited by R. Alexander, C. Doddington, J. Gray, L. Hargreaves and R. Kershner (Abingdon: Routledge, 2010) 49–82.
9   Tony Eaude, 'Creating Hospitable Space to Nurture Children's Spirituality – Possibilities and Dilemmas Associated with Power', *International Journal of Children's Spirituality* 19:3–4 (2014) 236-248, here 239 & 246.

David Csinos states that, 'educators, parents, pastors, and other adults can best nurture the spiritual lives of children by walking with them on the journey...[to] become co-learners with children in our quests to know God'. According to him, 'the adult should sometimes lead the child forward along the path... and at other moments the child should guide the adult as they seek together the presence of the living God'.[10] Coles also uses the image of the young pilgrim, 'well aware that life is a finite journey'.[11]

Possibly the best advice for adults who are accompanying children in the discovery of their spiritual selves and helping them make meaning from the existential questions that they encounter in life, comes from Rebecca Nye, who suggests that adults should talk less and listen more.

> ...habitually leaving longer gaps after a child had spoken in case they have more to say and allowing time for everyone to take in and value their contribution... instead of prematurely intruding into the auditory space when children have been speaking or planning to speak, adults can simply show their response and interest through facial expressions and 'mmms'.[12]

This is a tough skill; parents can have an inherent ability to master it, but perhaps other adults (teachers or chaplains) find difficulty with it. There is always the risk to provide the answer rather than giving encouragement to the questing and questioning mind of the child. From the apparent certainty of our adult worldview, it is easy to lapse into the habit of discounting the child's worldview and seeing it only as a rudimentary stage through which the child will go, but will eventually grow out of.

---

10 David M. Csinos, *Children's Ministry That Fits: Beyond One-size-Fits-all Approaches to Nurturing Children's Spirituality* (Eugene, OR: Wipf & Stock, 2011) 11–12.
11 Coles, *The Spiritual Life of Children*, xvi.
12 Nye, *Children's Spirituality*, 45.

Learning and celebrating in the domestic church

The pandemic seemed to be an appropriate time to focus on the concept of the domestic church. Within the confines of lockdown there was a great deal of consideration regarding the family. Parents became teachers and attempted to balance the care of their children with the commitments of working from home and working in the home – not only are reports compiled and deadlines met, but also meals are cooked, and the washing machine is on a continuous cycle. Children relied on the companionship of their siblings perhaps more than ever and learned to live in the confinement of houses and apartments without the regularity of school, sports or other activities. They had to contend themselves with Zoom and Skype encounters with beloved grandparents. This is the reality of the domestic church, the smallest unit within the Christian Church. As the Catechism states, we have the example of the Holy Family as model and inspiration and the practice of the entire family becoming believers in the early days of the Apostles.

> Christ chose to be born and grow up in the bosom of the holy family of Joseph and Mary. The Church is nothing other than 'the family of God'. From the beginning, the core of the Church was often constituted by those who had become believers 'together with all [their] household'. When they were converted, they desired that 'their whole household' should also be saved. These families who became believers were islands of Christian life in an unbelieving world.[13]

We called our first gatherings of Christians, 'house churches': followers gathered in each other's homes to celebrate and pray and be of mutual support to each other, both in times of sorrow and in times of joy.

---

13 *Catechism of the Catholic Church* (Dublin: Veritas, 1995), 1655.

The domestic church became a reality in twenty-first-century Ireland, as it had been a reality in the Ireland of the past. The Eucharist entered the domestic church in a particular way during lockdown – online. As people gathered around a laptop, phone or television, they prayed together. One parishioner told me that her teenage / adult children sat on the couch on Holy Saturday night, each watching the Easter Vigil on their own phone; teenagers who rarely attended in person, attended electronically – a novelty perhaps, but attend they did. In Ireland, at times when the Eucharist was absent or at best infrequent, the rosary was the staple of the domestic spiritual life. It served the purpose of prayer and spiritual communion, but also a moment of unity within the family. Loved ones who had died were remembered in the trimmings and the fate of family members who had emigrated was entrusted to the Heavenly Mother. As a practice it has all but died out; there are few families who gather for the family rosary in the way their parents and grandparents once did. This is a great pity, considering how much prayer the world needs at this time, and how much individuals and families have needed the consolation of prayer in coping with the stresses of the virus and the uncertainties that have come with it.

At the centre of this domestic church are the parents who, in fulfilment of the promise they made at the Baptism of their children, assume the role of first and best teachers in the ways of faith. This is laid out in the Constitution on the Church in the Modern World at the Second Vatican Council, 'The family is, so to speak, the domestic church. In it, parents should, by their word and example, be the first preachers of the faith to their children' (*Lumen Gentium*, 11). Parents have the ability to instil in their children the love of God and love of neighbour, and as the quotation says, they are called to do it by both word and example. In the child's life the role of teacher is important and likewise the role of the parish community, but they can never surpass the role of parents in catechesis. The Catechism goes on to reiterate the importance of the domestic Church: 'In our own time, in a world often alien and even hostile to faith, believing families are of primary importance as centres of living, radiant faith'. (CCC, 1656)

Within the domestic church there are still opportunities to teach children and occasions to draw out from them the seed of faith given at baptism. There are perhaps three distinct and interlinked aspects of this teaching. Firstly, there is the need to educate the children religiously. They do need the facts, the knowledge, the stories and the prayers. Religious education should help the children to grow in the knowledge of the person of Jesus Christ. Next is the catechetical dimension where we seek to form the children in faith and help them to take the lessons from religious education and put them into practice. Finally, there is sacramental preparation: the combination of religious education and catechesis and also the formation necessary for them to become part of the liturgical assembly and to be prepared for the reception of the sacraments, in particular First Holy Communion. The preparation for the sacraments in parishes has usually involved a sacramental preparation programme; in particular *Do This in Memory*. It has been a tremendous resource to parishes in attempting to bridge the gap between parish, home and school. However, most of these programmes were stopped in March 2020, and dates for their celebration generally passed in May and June without any of the celebrations happening.

Parents and the community of the family, in consideration of the aims of sacramental preparation, have options in the absence of a parish-based programme. *Directory for Masses with Children* states:

> All those who are concerned with education should work and plan together to ensure that the children, besides having some idea of God and the supernatural, should also, in proportion to their years and degree of maturity as persons, have experience of those human values which are involved in Eucharistic celebration: acting together as a community; exchanging greetings; the capacity to listen; to forgive and to

ask forgiveness; the expression of gratitude; the experience of symbolic actions, conviviality and festive celebration.[14]

It is the confluence of the 'human values' and the formation of the child which is paramount here, and what the child experiences will have a bearing on that formation. I frequently turn to this quotation when I am speaking to parents of children preparing for sacraments. These parents can often be intimidated by the prospect of contributing to the religious formation of their children, perhaps reflecting on their own inadequacies as people of faith. So, my first job is to assure them that all of us are inadequate when it comes to faith formation, but in the normal and everyday way that we 'live and move and have our being' (Acts 17:28) are the seeds of this formation, and the quotation from the *Directory for Masses with Children* is the key.

Parents are the first teachers in every way, not just in the ways of faith, as suggested by the Rite of Baptism. They teach them how to say 'please' and 'thank-you', when and how to say sorry, how to share their toys and how to be nice to others. Children understand the rituals of family very early on and they are certainly not reticent when it comes to celebrations. All these experiences of the child are what we bring to their gradual understanding of the celebration of the Eucharist. *Catechesi Tradendae* (CT), Pope John Paul II's letter on catechesis in our time, speaks of:

> ...a catechesis aimed at inserting him or her organically into the life of the Church, a moment that includes an immediate preparation for the celebration of the sacraments. It is a catechesis that gives meaning to the sacraments, but at the same time it receives from the experience of the sacraments a living dimension that keeps it from remaining merely doctrinal, and it communicates to the child the joy of being a witness to Christ in ordinary life. (CT, 37)

14 *Directory for Masses with Children*, 9

This can be formed in such a way as to allow this insertion into the life of the Church precisely because the children have been already inserted organically into the life of the family. There is no better time to bring home those 'human values' than when families are living in close quarters, and saying 'please', 'thank-you', and 'sorry' are so crucial to maintaining calm and positive wellbeing. In the absence of 'immediate preparation for the celebration of the sacraments,' the children can rely on learning not from the doctrinal dimensions, but from ordinary life.

During the pontificate of Benedict XVI and at a gathering of clergy in Bressanone in 2008, the Pope was asked a question regarding sacramental preparation and what seemed the futility of the endeavour considering the frequent lack of interest on the part of parents. This is an age-old question, but the Pope's answer was far from old. On the encounter with parents, he concluded,

> ...the pedagogy of faith is always a journey and we must accept today's situations. Yet, we must also open them more to each person, so that the result is not only an external memory of things that endures but that their hearts have truly been touched. The moment when we are convinced the heart is touched – it has felt a little of Jesus' love, it has felt a little the desire to move along these lines and in this direction. That is the moment when, it seems to me, we can say that we have made a true catechesis. The proper meaning of catechesis, in fact, must be this: to bring the flame of Jesus' love, even if it is a small one, to the hearts of children, and through the children to their parents, thus reopening the places of faith of our time.[15]

I think this time of pandemic has taught us many things; lessons, perhaps, that we were not eager or ready to learn. It can also teach

---

15 Pope Benedict, 'Meeting of the Holy Father Benedict XVI with the clergy of the diocese of Bolzano-Bressanone', Holy See Press Office, www.vatican.va/content/benedict-xvi/en.speeches/2008/august/document/ hf-benxvi_spe_20080806_clero-bressanone.html.

parents the value and grace of not only accompanying their children in their faith journey, but also seeing this fundamental task of parenthood as intrinsic to their own faith journey – becoming aware of the spiritual nature of children and how that nature is intrinsically part of them, just like every other aspect of their being. Helping the children to give voice to their imaginings of God, to their questions about life and its meaning, to their hopes and aspirations for the future and for their fears and anxieties in the present, will bring a richness to the life of both parent and child. Pope Benedict was telling the audience that when the heart of the child is opened to catechesis and when a child's spiritual life is nurtured by that catechesis, it will always have a reverberation into the heart and soul of the parent.

Questions for Reflection and Discussion

1. During the months of pandemic restrictions, what elements of religious formation have children missed out on?
2. During these months, what elements of religious formation have children gained?
3. How can a family become a domestic church in the reality of daily life?
4. In your experience, what can children teach adults about God and spirituality?

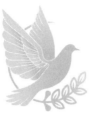

Catholic Social Teaching and COVID-19

Pádraig Corkery

*O*ver the past twelve months, an amount has been written and spoken about the pandemic and its impact on individuals, communities, and economies. This global event has raised fundamental questions about, among other things, human vulnerability and the nature of the bonds that tie people together as families, communities and societies. The disciplines of anthropology, sociology and psychology have been busy grappling with these fundamental questions. The Catholic tradition has also reflected deeply on the pandemic and the questions it raises about God and the nature of Christian identity and worship. These discussions are to be found in pastoral letters, in homilies and in theological journals.[1] For an ecumenical approach to the pandemic see the thought-provoking joint publication by the Pontifical Council for Interreligious Dialogue (PCID) and the World Council of Churches (WCC).[2] In this

---

1 To take the example of just one Irish journal, see Eamon Fitzgibbon, 'Pastoral Practice in this Time', *The Furrow* 71 (July/August 2020): 396–403; Michael Neary, 'Covid-19 – A Challenge to Faith', *The Furrow* 71 (September 2020): 455–458; Brendan Leahy, 'Ten Covid-19 "Outcomes" for the Church', *The Furrow* 71 (May 2020): 285–291; Kevin Hargaden, 'Killing for the Eucharist', *The Furrow* 71 (September 2020): 459–465; Richard Scriven, 'Placing Pilgrimage during Covid-19', *The Furrow* 71 (July/August 2020): 404–410.

2 Pontifical Council for Interreligious Dialogue and the World Council of Churches, *Serving a Wounded World in Interreligious Solidarity: A Christian Call to Reflection and Action During COVID-19 and Beyond*. This document can be downloaded at www.cwmission.org/wp-content/uploads/2020/12/Serving-a-wounded-world-in-interreligious-solidarity.pdf. .

article they bring the Christian understanding of human existence into creative conversation with the reality and implications of COVID-19.[3]

Very obviously the pandemic has highlighted our shared humanity and, especially, our vulnerability and mutual dependence. No one is immune from the virus and the upheavals that accompany it. Suffering, fear, loss and death are universally experienced. The limitations on our freedoms as a consequence of the pandemic have caused anger, loss and frustration. This is especially true of those who were unable to journey with a loved one in their final days. Or those who were unable to celebrate positive and joyful family events in a manner that we have grown accustomed to. The reality of our interdependence is the foundation on which people have worked together to try and limit the spread of the virus.[4]

I think it is true to say that the pandemic has the potential to reveal important truths about what it means to be a member of the human family. Such truths were often ignored or undervalued when we were living in a more stable time of easy travel, dining experiences without time constraints and social engagements that were mask-free. How we understand the human person is decisive because it shapes how we relate to self, others, creation and the Transcendent. There are fundamental questions relating to our origin, destiny and freedom that all persons feel driven to engage with. Are we rugged individuals or are we social by nature? Are there limits to human freedom? What is the goal or meaning of human existence? Recent Catholic teaching has emphasised that the many moral issues burdening humanity – war, hatred, exploitation, new forms of human slavery, ecological degradation, dehumanising poverty – are not disconnected but are, rather, linked. They often flow from a particular [flawed] understanding of the roots and content of human dignity, the scope of human freedom, and the nature of human destiny[5].

---

3   For a succinct reflection on this document see Kevin O'Gorman, 'Serving a Wounded World', *The Furrow* 71 (October 2020): 575–578.

4   Michael Sandel, 'The Tablet Interview', *The Tablet*, 5 September 2020, p. 11.

5   See, for example, Pope Francis, *Laudato Si'* (Dublin: Veritas, 2015) Chapter 3.

Christian anthropology

The Christian family has over the centuries articulated its own understanding of the human person that is rooted in revelation, reason and the living tradition of a faith community. Central to this understanding is the claim that we are, all of us, created in God's image (Gen 1:27). The implications of this bold claim are manifold and profound; our dignity is intrinsic to us – it flows from our reality as sons and daughters of God and is not dependent on our achievements, virtue, health, race or social standing; there is a Godly or spiritual dimension to our existence – we are not one-dimensional persons who can be satisfied by 'bread alone'; our destiny is linked to our origin – we come from God and we ultimately rest in God. Furthermore, Revelation presents Christ as the model for humanity and for Christian discipleship. Hence the actions and words of Christ should shape the world-view, attitudes and actions of the disciple. Engagement with self, others, creation and the Transcendent should be marked by respect, awe, justice, compassion and a spirit of thankfulness.

Catholic social doctrine

The implication of this anthropology, revealed in Scripture, is continually being teased out in the living tradition of the Church and most particularly in the Catholic Social Doctrine tradition.[6] This tradition, beginning with Leo XIII's encyclical *Rerum Novarum* (1891), brings the light of the Gospel to bear on the nature of the societies we construct. It scrutinises the political, economic and social policies created by societies to ensure that such policies respect human dignity, promote justice and inclusion, care for the vulnerable and respect the integrity of creation. Integral to Catholic Social Teaching is an optimism that we can create societies that are inclusive, just and peaceful, and better reflect the values of the Gospel.

This dimension of the Church's living tradition also proposes core principles to guide individuals and faith communities in the process

---

6   For an accessible overview of the content and history of Catholic Social Teaching see Kenneth R. Himes, ed., *Modern Catholic Social Teaching: Commentaries and Interpretations*, 2nd edition (Washington, DC: Georgetown University Press, 2018).

of discernment that leads to action. Often referred to as the 'Church's best kept secret' this corpus of teaching is at the core of any authentic Catholic identity. Indeed, a much quoted paragraph from the Synod of Bishops in 1971 stated that 'action on behalf of justice and participation in the transformation of the world fully appear to us as a constitutive dimension of the preaching of the Gospel, or, in other words, of the Church's mission for the redemption of the human race and its liberation from every oppressive situation.'[7] Furthermore, the *Compendium of the Social Doctrine of the Church* (CSDC) states quite categorically that 'insofar as it is part of the Church's moral teaching, the Church's social doctrine has the same dignity and authority as her moral teaching. It is authentic Magisterium, which obligates the faithful to adhere to it' (CSDC, 80).

The Church's social teaching highlights an essential dimension of the Christian life: its *oneness*. Right belief (orthodoxy) leads to right living (orthopraxis). We are called, in the language of the Gospel, to be the 'salt of the earth' and 'the light of the world' (Mt 5:13–14). Hence, we are called to allow the values of the Gospel to shape our own lives and the societies we participate in and help construct or maintain through our choices (political and otherwise), actions and attitudes. The *oneness* of the Christian life was emphasised with great clarity by Pope John Paul II in *Christifideles Laici*, his 1988 letter on the vocation and mission of the lay faithful in the Church and the world. There he argued that for Christians there cannot 'be two parallel lives in their existence: on the one hand, the so-called 'spiritual' life with its values and demands, and on the other the so-called 'secular' life, that is life in a family, at work, in social relationships, in the responsibilities of public life and in culture'.[8] For the believer there is only one life, an integrated life where our faith shapes how we respond to those who people our lives and especially those on the margins.

---

7   Synod of Bishops, *Justice in the World* (Vatican City: Pontifical Commission for Justice and Peace, 1972–1973), 6.

8   John Paul II, *Christifideles Laici* (Vatican City: Libreria Editrice Vaticana, 1988), 59. See also the *Compendium*, 546.

The COVID-19 pandemic

The importance of Catholic Social Teaching and its relevance to the current pandemic was highlighted by Pope Francis in the autumn of 2020 when he dedicated his Wednesday General Audiences to the principles and insights of that tradition. He strongly argued that Catholic Social Teaching offers a valuable set of principles for world leaders navigating the economic and social havoc caused by the pandemic. This theme is further developed in his 2020 encyclical *Fratelli Tutti*. What, then, are these principles?

The *Compendium* lists *five* principles that direct the Church's engagement with and commentary on the economic, social and political spheres. The five principles are: the common good, the universal destination of the world's goods, solidarity, subsidiarity and participation. These principles are informed and directed by three fundamental values: truth, freedom and justice. The principles themselves do not work in isolation but must rather 'be appreciated in their unity, interrelatedness and articulation' (CSDC, 162). The application of these value-driven principles to a particular context involves discernment and a prudential judgement. The *end* to which these principles are directed is the creation of societies that enable human flourishing by being just, caring, inclusive, free and respectful of the integrity of creation. Or to put it another way: societies that respect and protect the truth of *who we are.*

The principle of the *common good* is particularly relevant to our recent pandemic-shaped reality. The language of the common good has been employed daily in the directives and advice issued by Ireland's National Public Health Emergency Team (NPHET) and a range of other government agencies. In a well-received pastoral letter in the 1990s the Bishops of England and Wales urged voters to vote for candidates that best promoted and protected the common good.[9] What, then, is the common good and how can it be promoted

---

9   Catholic Bishops' Conference of England and Wales, *The Common Good and the Catholic Church's Social Teaching* (Manchester: Gabriel Communications, 1996). The global dimension of the common good is highlighted in a pastoral letter of the Irish Episcopal Conference, *Towards the Global Common Good* (Dublin: Veritas, 2005).

in these pandemic times?[10] The Second Vatican Council's document *Gaudium et Spes* (GS) understood the common good as 'the sum total of social conditions which allow people, either as groups or as individuals, to reach their fulfilment more fully and more easily' (GS, 26). This definition has stood the test of time and has appeared in later Church teaching documents.

Catholic Social Teaching argues that political and economic activity in society should be directed towards, and be under the judgement of, the common good rather than being guided by sectional interests that, inevitably, lead to marginalisation and exclusion.[11] If human fulfilment is the goal of economic and political activity, then such activity must include the *whole* person and *every* person. It cannot be reduced to economic progress only, but must include in its remit all the elements that enable persons to reach their potential. These include, but are not limited to, access to quality health care and education, peace and stability, equal and fair treatment before the law, access to work and to healthy and safe work environments, religious freedom and respect for the rights of conscience. The inclusion of the right to religious freedom is important because, if the common good is truly directed towards the good or end of the human person, it cannot 'be deprived of its transcendent dimension' (CSDC, 170). In recent decades we have discovered a greater sense of the interconnected nature of all of creation and so the common good has a necessary *global* dimension. The consequences of economic and political activity must be evaluated from the perspective of the global community – how does it impact on the lives of those in less developed countries and, indeed, on our shared environment and home?

During the COVID pandemic the notion of the common good was invoked to restrict our freedoms in many different zones of human activity including travel, celebrations of weddings and funerals, access to education, visitations to loved ones in hospitals and other

---

10 For a concise account of the common good and the other key principles, see Chapter 4 of the *Compendium*. For a more scholarly study see Patrick Riordan, *A Grammar of the Common Good* (London: Continuum, 2008).

11 See Pope Francis, *Evangelii Gaudium*, 53–54 (No to an economy of exclusion), 55–56 (No to the new idolatry of money), 57–58 (No to a financial system which rules rather than serves).

care facilities. The vast majority of people accepted this limitation on their freedom as proportionate and necessary in order to protect the common good of Irish society and the global common good.[12]

Solidarity is another important principle of the Catholic Social Teaching tradition that is relevant to our contemporary context. The roots of the principle of solidarity are to be found in our shared humanity, the equality of persons and our nature as social beings. *Solidarity* is also understood as a virtue that, like all the virtues, disposes us towards acting in a particular fashion and shapes our character. The content of this principle and virtue was powerfully unpacked by Pope John Paul II in his encyclical *Sollicitudo Rei Socialis* (1987, SRS).[13] Solidarity, he suggested, is 'not a feeling of vague compassion or shallow distress at the misfortunes of so many people, both near and far. On the contrary, it is a firm and persevering determination to commit oneself to the common good – that is to say, the good of all and of each individual, because we are all really responsible for all' (SRS, 38).

The implications of solidarity for a community fighting the pandemic are many – journeying with those who are sick and vulnerable; supporting those working on the frontline; working together as communities in a coordinated and single-minded fashion; praying together for, amongst other things, the guidance and wisdom of the Holy Spirit.

The third principle of the social teaching tradition that is relevant to our current context is that of the *universal destination of the world's goods* (CSDC, 171–184). This principle states boldly that God made the world for everyone and that all have a *right* to benefit from the fruits of creation. Moreover, this right is 'a natural right, inscribed in human nature and not merely a positive right, --- [It] is innate in individual persons, in every person' (CSDC, 172). This princi-

---

12   For an interesting new book on the challenges to the notion of the common good see Michael Sandel, *The Tyranny of Merit: What's Become of the Common Good?* (London: Allen Lane, 2020).

13   Pope John Paul II, *Sollicitudo Rei Socialis*, www.vatican.va/content/john-paul-ii/en/encyclicals/documents/hf_jp-ii_enc_30121987_sollicitudo-rei-socialis.html.

ple relativizes the right to private property and directs political and economic activity towards the realisation of the principle: 'All other rights, whatever they are, including property rights and the right of free trade, must be subordinated to this norm (the universal destination of goods); they must not hinder it, but must rather expedite its application' (CSDC, 172).[14] This is a very radical principle that raises very important questions for all societies, including Ireland. The implications of this principle include universal access to health care, education, work, housing[15] and the right to appropriate subsidies that are necessary for the subsistence of unemployed workers and their families (CSDC, 301). It is also a principle that informs some of the Catholic reflection on the Universal Basic Income debate.

The decision of the Government in 2020 to assist the many thousands whose employment ceased during the pandemic and their making available universal free COVID testing is a fine example of this principle in action. But it is a principle that should continue to unsettle us because of its implications for the policies and choices we pursue in housing, healthcare, education and remuneration. If we compare nurses or caregivers with lawyers or accountants, the vast difference in remuneration rates in Ireland and other 'developed' economies is worth reflecting on in light of this principle and also in light of the teaching of Pope John Paul II that the sources of the dignity of work 'are to be sought primarily in the subjective dimension, not in the objective one'.[16] Work has value primarily because it is a *person* who does the work.

The current pandemic has brought with it suffering, death and the disruption of the 'normal' patterns of living and relating. It has also impacted negatively on the local and global economies and put the brakes on many projects of expansion and innovation because of uncertainty about the future. It has highlighted fundamental truths about humanity – our vulnerability, our equality, our nature as social

---

14   See Paul VI, *Populorum Progressio* (London: CTS, 1967), #22.
15   For a challenging document on access to housing see the Irish Catholic Bishops' Conference, *A Room at the Inn: A Pastoral Letter on Housing and Homelessness* (Dublin: Veritas, 2017).
16   Pope John Paul II, *Laborem Exercens* (Dublin: Veritas, 1981), 6.

beings and our interdependence. The response to the pandemic in Ireland and elsewhere has been, by and large, one of shared effort, solidarity with one another and care for the vulnerable. For believers, this is a response that is mandated by the call of the Gospel and the nature of Christian discipleship. This response can be enriched and enlightened by the foundations and content of Catholic Social Teaching as we journey through these challenging times.

Questions for Reflection and Discussion

1. In practical terms, what can we do to promote the common good in these difficult times?
2. In your experience, what challenges to human solidarity have been posed by the COVID-19 pandemic?
3. How can we ensure that the social and economic impact of COVID-19 on the most vulnerable is limited?
4. Which important truths has the pandemic revealed about what it means to be human?

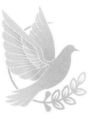

Encountering God's Mercy in Extraordinary Times: Celebrating the Sacrament of Reconciliation during a Pandemic

Michael Mullaney

Every dimension of life has been disrupted and disorientated by COVID-19. Public health restrictions on gatherings in churches, social / physical distancing requirements, sanitisation and hygiene measures have created severe impediments, or made it even impossible for the faithful participating in the 'ordinary' celebration of the sacraments. While live-streamed or online celebrations of the sacraments are no substitute for that profound experience of God which only the living, liturgical and sacramental life of the Church can offer, the internet has provided a virtual lifeline for many parish communities through the turmoil of 'lockdown'.

The on-going public health guidance continues to pose particular challenges for the celebration of the Sacrament of Reconciliation. Some churches have notices announcing that the Sacrament of Reconciliation is not available at this time; and where the faithful can approach the sacrament, it is not always possible to ensure the due precautions of distancing between the priest and the faithful. During a national or county 'lockdown', the restrictions on travel make individual confession even more difficult.

In this exceptional and extraordinary time of a global pandemic, the Church can avail of the exceptional and extraordinary means at its disposal in canon law to ensure the right of the baptised to experience and encounter God's grace, mercy and healing communicated in the sacramental life of the Church. In this context, it is worth reflecting on a *Note from the Apostolic Penitentiary on the Sacrament of Penance in the current pandemic situation* (henceforth: *The Note*), issued by the Vatican on 20 March 2020, that ensures that in this 'time of poverty' God's mercy can still reach us in extraordinary ways.

It is useful to reaffirm important fundamental principles of canonical doctrine in relation to the sacraments before looking at the celebration of the Sacrament of Reconciliation during a pandemic. There are two key reasons for the Church's regulation (canon law) of the sacraments. First is the right of the baptised to receive the sacraments, and the second is the obligation of the minister to celebrate them in conformity with their nature; that is, as Christ intended them. The first, the right to the sacraments, can be found in the combined provisions in canons 213 and 843, §1. On the one hand: 'Christ's faithful have a right to be assisted by their pastors from the spiritual riches of the Church, especially by the Word of God and the sacraments' (Can. 213). However, every right necessitates a corresponding obligation in order to be realised: 'Sacred ministers may not deny the sacraments to those who opportunely ask for them, are properly disposed and are not prohibited by law from receiving them' (Can. 843, §1).[1]

The second reason, the obligation to celebrate the sacraments in conformity to their nature, is rooted in the doctrine that Christ entrusted the sacraments to the Church: 'As actions of Christ and of the Church, they are signs and means by which faith is expressed and strengthened, worship offered to God and our sanctification is brought about. Thus, they contribute in the most effective manner to establishing, strengthening and manifesting ecclesiastical commu-

---

1   The Canon Law Society of Great Britain and Ireland, *The Code of Canon Law in English Translation* (London: Collins, 1983).

nion' (Can. 840). The Church, therefore, is bound to obey the mandate of Christ and remain faithful to what Christ has instituted. This ensures that the sign (word and action) is not subject to the discretion of the minister or the community, but protected and guarded by the Church for the realisation of salvation.

However, in the celebration of the sacraments, the Church has always had the power to establish and change that which it judges necessary to respond to changing times, circumstances and places, for the benefit of those who receive them: 'Since the sacraments are the same throughout the universal Church, and belong to the divine deposit of faith, only the supreme authority in the Church can approve or define what is needed for their validity. It belongs to the same authority, or another competent authority in accordance with can. 838, §§ 3 and 4, to determine what is required for their lawful celebration, administration and reception and for the order to be observed in their celebration' (Can. 841). It should be noted that the canon speaks of 'supreme authority' as regards the requirements of validity, thus highlighting the intimate connection between the celebration of the sacraments and the unity of the Church. It is of 'the same authority or other competent authority', to determine the conditions of lawfulness and the liturgical rite. However, this competence is not left unspecified, because the canon identifies them: the Apostolic See, Episcopal Conferences, and Diocesan Bishops.

On 20 March 2020, the Apostolic Penitentiary issued *The Note* because 'the gravity of the present circumstances calls for reflection on the urgency and centrality of the Sacrament of Reconciliation, together with some necessary clarifications, both for the lay faithful and for ministers called to celebrate the Sacrament'.

Individual and integral confession
Individual and integral confession is affirmed in *The Note* as the ordinary way of celebrating the Sacrament of Reconciliation. Physical and moral impossibility alone excuses from such confessions, in which case reconciliation may be attained by other means too (Can.

960). Individual and integral confession requires on the part of the penitent the disposition of sincere contrition, confession of sins, purpose of amendment; on the part of the priest, absolution.

Some priests have met the challenge of providing individual and integral confession by celebrating the Sacrament of Reconciliation in church car parks or organising 'drive-in' confessions where the penitent sits in their car and the priest sits at the prescribed distance from the car window, wearing the necessary protective materials (such as PPE, facemasks or visors) and with a screen to protect the identity of the penitent. Prudent measures need to be adopted in the individual celebration of sacramental reconciliation, such as holding the celebration in a ventilated place outside the confessional, the adoption of a suitable distance, the use of protective masks, without prejudice to absolute attention to the safeguarding of the sacramental seal and the necessary discretion.

The document issued in June 2020 by the Irish Episcopal Conference, *Framework Document for the Public Return to the Celebration of Mass and the Sacraments*, echoes the guidance of *The Note* and affirms that the celebration of the sacraments must be balanced with the requirement that 'in all circumstances the safety and health of people, ministers, and priests must be paramount'.[2] With regard to the Sacrament of Reconciliation, the framework document states that 'provision should be made in the body of the Church for a confessional area. Consideration should be given to the privacy of the sacrament as well as the requirements of physical distancing and hygiene'. For any individual and integral celebration of the Sacrament of Reconciliation during this pandemic, priests should take maximum care and be equipped with a suitable protective mask and, where possible, with mutual health protection devices (e.g. PPE).

---

2   Irish Catholic Bishops' Conference, 'Statement of the Irish Catholic Bishops' Conference on the publication of the Framework Document for a return to the public celebration of Mass and the Sacraments', 9/06/20, www.catholicbishops.ie/2020/06/09/statement-of-the-irish-catholic-bishops-conference-on-the-publication-of-the-framework-document-for-a-return-to-the-public-celebration-of-mass-and-the-sacraments.

General absolution

The Apostolic Penitentiary permits the use of general or collective absolution in certain situations. While outlining the canonical discipline that collective or general absolution cannot be imparted except where there is an imminent danger of death or grave necessity (Can. 961, § 1), *The Note* permits for the period of health emergency that the priests and religious appointed by the bishop can give absolution to several penitents without prior individual confession when the sick or hospitalised are in danger of death or are in wards where it is not possible to guarantee adequate measures to avoid contagion. Absolution can also be given to health personnel who request it.

The two requirements for general absolution, 'danger of death' and 'grave necessity', are both present during a pandemic. The primary recipients of the intervention are the infected faithful in danger of death. With regard to the manner of the general absolution, *The Note* requires the minister of the sacrament to observe as much as possible the personalistic character or context of the sacrament. The personalistic dimension is underlined by specifying where the minister should be when giving general absolution: 'the entrance to hospital wards where there are infected faithful who are in danger of death, using as much as possible and with the necessary precautions, means of vocal amplification so that the absolution may be heard'. This may be modified so that absolution is given in a way that those present can hear the words of the priest, respecting as much as possible, the sensitivities of non-believers or those who are non-Christian. Penitents are in some way to be advised, if possible, of the conditions for receiving absolution: repentance for their sins and the intention to confess serious ones when, once the current circumstances are overcome or health is restored, individual confession can be accessed.

The question arises if there are any other scenarios in which general absolution could be given during a pandemic? Shortly after *The Note* was issued by the Apostolic Penitentiary, Pope Francis recalled a conversation he had with an Italian bishop in an interview with the journalist Austen Ivereigh, reprinted in this book:

About a week ago an Italian bishop, somewhat flustered, called me. He had been going around the hospitals wanting to give absolution to those inside the wards from the hallway of the hospital. But he had spoken to canon lawyers who had told him he couldn't, that absolution could only be given in direct contact. 'What do you think, Holy Father?' he had asked me. I told him: 'Bishop, fulfil your priestly duty.' And the bishop said '*Grazie, ho capito*' ('Thank you, I understand'). I found out later that he was giving absolution all around the place. This is the freedom of the Spirit in the midst of a crisis, not a Church closed off in institutions. That doesn't mean that canon law is not important: it is, it helps, and please let's make good use of it, it is for our good. But the final canon says that the whole of canon law is for the salvation of souls, and that's what opens the door for us to go out in times of difficulty to bring the consolation of God.

What of the possibility of general absolution if there were to be another significant surge or substantial spike in the number affected by the pandemic contagion and further restrictions in travel? Is there is a possibility that a diocesan bishop after reviewing the criteria agreed upon with the other members of the Episcopal Conference (cf. Can. 455, § 2) could authorise the celebration of general absolution, to avoid the risk of infection for people and priests? But even any gathering of people for the celebration of general absolution during this pandemic is fraught with risk. *The Note* offers a further exceptional way to encounter God's mercy: perfect contrition.

Perfect contrition

In his daily meditation on 20 March 2020, Pope Francis referred to the act of perfect contrition: 'If you don't find a priest to go to Confession, speak to God. He is your Father. Tell him the truth: "Lord. I did this and this and this. Pardon me." Ask his forgiveness with all your heart with an Act of Contrition, and promise him, "afterward I will go to Confession, but forgive me now." You will return to God's grace immediately. You yourself can draw near to God's forgiveness, as the Catechism teaches us, without having a priest at hand. Think about it: this is the moment! This is the right moment, the appropriate moment. An Act of Contrition, made well. In this way our souls will become as white as snow.'

The reference Pope Francis made to perfect contrition in the *Catechism of the Catholic Church* is found in paragraphs 1451–52: 'Among the penitent's acts contrition occupies first place. Contrition is 'sorrow of the soul and detestation for the sin committed, together with the resolution not to sin again'. When it arises from a love by which God is loved above all else, contrition is called "perfect" (contrition of charity). Such contrition remits venial sins; it also obtains forgiveness of mortal sins if it includes the firm resolution to have recourse to sacramental Confession as soon as possible'. A theological principle of St Thomas Aquinas, taken up from Peter Lombard, is also present in the *Code of Canon Law* (1257): 'God has bound salvation to the Sacrament of Baptism, but God is not bound by the sacraments.' This can also be applied to the Sacrament of Reconciliation. It is the doctrine of the 'sacrament of desire'. It is a humble reminder that the sacraments do not belong to us, but to Christ and a powerful reminder of the extraordinary ends to which God the Father will go to embrace us in his mercy.

The *Note* of the Apostolic Penitentiary also affirms: 'Where individual faithful may be in the painful impossibility of receiving sacramental absolution, it should be remembered that perfect contrition, coming from the love of God, loved above all else, expressed by a sincere request for forgiveness (one which the penitent is able to express in that moment) and accompanied by the *votum confessionis*, that is, by the firm resolution to receive sacramental Confession as soon as possible, obtains the forgiveness of sins, even mortal ones (cf. CCC, 1452)'. In the face of sincere and profound repentance, it is therefore possible, in this extraordinary time, to receive God's forgiveness, by committing oneself to approach the Sacrament of Reconciliation as soon as the situation permits.

Confession via phone/online

The question has been posed during the pandemic whether it is possible to hear a confession and impart absolution by telephone or on-line. The question is understandable given the widespread use and easy access to online communications. There is an historical precedent for the question, the so-called 'confessions from a distance' query regarding the possibility of confessing and receiving absolution by letter. Not surprisingly, the Holy Office responded negatively at the time. The question surfaced again with the appearance of the telephone. Again, the magisterium was not favourable to this, explaining that the spread of such a practice would contradict the 'social dimension' of the sacrament which has a strong ecclesial and liturgical aspect, and would ultimately lead to a privatisation of Confession.

The arrival of the internet and online meetings has given fresh impetus to the question. Writing on the occasion of the 36th World Communications Day (24 January 2002) in the document *Internet: A New Forum for Proclaiming the Gospel* (n. 3), Pope John Paul II wrote: 'The Internet can never replace that profound experience of God which only the living, liturgical and sacramental life of the Church can offer'.[3] This was reaffirmed in a document from the Pontifical Council for Social Communications, *The Church and the Internet* (n. 9) which stated: 'Virtual reality is no substitute for the Real Presence of Christ in the Eucharist, the sacramental reality of the other sacraments, and shared worship in a flesh-and-blood human community. There are no sacraments on the Internet; and even the religious experiences possible there by the grace of God are insufficient apart from real-world interaction with other persons of faith'.[4]

A major concern with the use of the phone or the internet in the celebration of the Sacrament of Reconciliation, however, even when public health guidelines require priests and penitents to maintain

3   Pope John Paul II, 'Message of the Holy Father John Paul II for the 36th World Communications Day', Holy See Press Office, 12/05/02, http://www.vatican.va/content/john-paul-ii/en/messages/communications/documents/hf_jp-ii_mes_20020122_world-communications-day.html.

4   Pontifical Council for Social Communications, 'The Church and the Internet', Holy See Press Office, http://www.vatican.va/roman_curia/pontifical_councils/pccs/documents/rc_pc_pccs_doc_20020228_church-internet_en.html.

social distancing, is the protection of the seal of confession. Today, this protection cannot be guaranteed online. Beyond this risk, however, the real issue is the undermining of the personalistic character and context of the celebration of the Sacrament of Reconciliation. Personal dialogue between the penitent and the confessor is essential. Confession brings the penitent into personal closeness with Christ in the person of the priest. Once again, the question of the use of the phone or Confession online because of the physical unavailability of a confessor already has a solution presented in *The Note*: an act of perfect contrition until the opportunity arrives for the sacrament itself.

Ordinarily, God's grace and mercy heals the wounds of sin and restores the bonds of communion through the individual and integral confession, but in extraordinary times, no one can prevent God from reaching us by extraordinary ways. As for the Sacrament of Reconciliation, the tradition of the Church indicates two of them: general absolution and the perfect act of contrition. Both Pope Francis (in his daily meditation of 20 March 2020 in Santa Marta) and *The Note* of the Apostolic Penitentiary confirm them. The sacraments are not magical gestures, which automatically produce grace, and they cannot be celebrated except in a real and not a virtual or digital presence. In the current pandemic, we can be open to extraordinary ways for God's mercy to receive us.

Questions for Reflection and Discussion

1. In your locality, how easy or difficult has it been to access individual confession?
2. During the pandemic, have you experienced any situation where you feel that general absolution could have been considered?
3. How aware are we as Catholics that perfect contrition is enough for God's forgiveness when sacramental Confession is impossible?
4. What are the benefits and limitations of the internet for the Church's liturgical prayers?

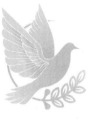

Praying in a Time of Pandemic

Kevin O'Gorman, SMA

'Deliver, Lord, your Church, to save it from all evil.'
(First / second century *Didache* 10)

'In liturgy as in life, the stakes are high.'[1]

*J*ust prior to the outbreak of the COVID-19 crisis, a copy of Bishop B. C. Butler's book *Prayer*[2] came to hand. As the pandemic intensified and increasingly became the sole topic of conversation in society and the media, the book's subtitle – *An Adventure in Living* – raised serious questions for 'prayer and faith' in a period that focussed on sheer survival. The title of two popular songs from the 1970s – 'Stayin' Alive' (The Bee Gees) and 'Surviving the Life' (Neil Diamond) – sounded more in tune with the time and its troubles. The second phrase in the latter's lyrics, 'Providing the soul', presents the problem of survival not solely in physical but also in spiritual terms. The 'terms and conditions' of lockdown and separation raised issues of both health, arising from illness, and hope as a result of isolation.

In the Foreword of his book Butler speaks of 'ordinary unassuming

---

1   Nathan Mitchell, 'The Amen Corner: Wrestling with the Word,' *Worship* 66/5 (September 1992), 465. Quoted in Gabe Huck, ed., *A Sourcebook about Liturgy*, (Chicago: Liturgy Training Publications, 1994), 161.
2   B. C. Butler, *Prayer* (London: Catholic Truth Society, 1983).

busy folk faced, as we all are, by the immeasurable mystery of existence and the need to take up some position in the face of that mystery'.[3] The global experience of the pandemic has engendered existential and economic, ethical and evangelical questions for many of us, if not all, as we are forced to face assumptions about so-called 'normal living'. Opening up the scope of his work Butler offers the following invitation: 'But I would hope that even an agnostic, if this book should fall into his hands, would catch some glimpse of the meaning which it tries to express, and would judge it no betrayal of his intellectual integrity to feel that it would be good if these things could be found to be true'.[4] Appealing to integrity, prayer in a time of pandemic seeks to identify, interpret and intercede for 'these things'.

The Embolism, the prayer immediately following the Lord's Prayer in the Communion Rite of the Mass, offers an opportunity to both explore and express the things essential to human survival on earth. Described in the *General Instruction of the Roman Missal* as 'developing the last petition of the Lord's Prayer itself, [it] asks for deliverance from the power of evil for the whole community of the faithful'.[5] Placed between the Our Father and the doxology, the Embolism is an expression of both petition and proclamation. Ending on an eschatological note, it can be extended to embrace the whole of humanity in its explicit reference to the Second Coming of Christ the Redeemer. As an elucidation of 'prayer and faith' in and for a time of emergency, the Embolism is eminently eloquent.

Deliver us, Lord, we pray, from every evil
Deliverance has a deep biblical resonance, beginning with the release of Israel from bondage in Egypt. This deliverance is the basis of their bond as a people under the leadership of Moses and their belonging to God by covenant. Daniel Harrington declares that 'what was new about the Mosaic religion was the emphasis on the escape from Egypt

---

3   Butler, *Prayer*, 10.
4   Ibid.
5   *The Roman Missal*, (Dublin: Veritas, 2011), xlii, no. 81.

as the great act of God on behalf of his people'.[6] Deliverance is a dynamic description of God's intervention in the life of both Israel and individuals. Despite hearing 'so many disparaging me, "Terror from every side! Denounce him!"' the prophet Jeremiah proclaims he will sing and praise 'the Lord for he has delivered the soul of the needy from the hands of evil persons' (Jer 20:10, 13). The Psalmist issues the poetic petition, 'Deliver us, O Lord, from our bondage as streams in dry land' (Ps 126[125]:4). Detailing the distinctiveness of divine deliverance in the Old Testament and describing its many different deeds, Wilhelm Kasch declares that 'they are determined by the creating and sustaining will of Yahweh for whom the salvation of the people and the individual is part of his creative action in the salvation history commenced by him. Because he is the sovereign Lord of this history, the nature, range and possibility of deliverance are wholly dependent on him and his will'.[7]

Although the idea of deliverance is central to the proclamation of the New Testament, the English versions of the NT vary in their wording to express this theme. One important passage occurs in Luke 4:18, where Jesus sets out his mission in the synagogue at Nazareth, quoting from Isaiah. Raymond Brown comments that 'the passage (Is 61:1–2), which reflects the Jubilee-year amnesty for the oppressed, is used to portray Jesus as an anointed prophet and is programmatic of what Jesus' 'ministry will bring about'.[8] Whereas the *King James Version* translates the third part of this programme as 'to preach deliverance to the captives', many other versions refer to 'release' rather than 'deliverance'. Whatever the exact translation here, the Bible employs a variety of synonyms to teach that God is a God of deliverance. In his letters, Paul places Christ at the centre of God's plan for deliverance of humanity from evil, declaring that the Father 'has rescued us from the power of darkness and transferred us into

---

6   Daniel Harrington, *Interpreting the Old Testament* (Wilmington, DE: Michael Glazier, 1981), 28.
7   Wilhelm Kasch, '*ruomai*', in Gerhard Kittel, ed., *Theological Dictionary of the New Testament*, Volume VI (Grand Rapids, MI: Eerdmans, 1968) 998-1003, here 1001.
8   Raymond Brown, *Introduction to the New Testament* (New York: Doubleday, 1997), 237.

the kingdom of his beloved Son' (Col 1:13 NRSV). With universal deliverance ultimately dependent on the death and resurrection of Jesus, Luke depicts its delivery on earth in the deeds of Jesus during his public ministry. As John Navone notes, 'the characteristically Lucan theme of salvation' is 'linked with *deliverance from death* in the account about Jairus' daughter' and 'associated with deliverance from diabolical possession; and with the remission of sins in the case of the sinful woman and Zacchaeus'.[9]

Illness and isolation, sickness and separation are among the physical and social evils experienced by people during the pandemic. The daily register of cases and deaths reported both at home and abroad have made for sombre statistics. One letter writer thanked the medical and scientific community for 'the reintroduction of the word "death" into common parlance', instead of 'the dreaded Americanism "passed away" or more commonly, and worse, "passed" to describe what happens when a body breathes its last'.[10] The prevalence of deaths and the poignancy of restricted funeral rites due to the pandemic drive the need for deliverance from this dreaded form of evil, drawing down prayer that the coronavirus may pass. Acknowledging the reality of death in this life, the Second Vatican Council affirmed that 'while the imagination is at a loss before the mystery of death, the Church, taught by divine revelation, declares that God has created people in view of a blessed destiny that lies beyond the boundaries of earthly misery'.[11] Praying to be delivered from 'every evil', especially in the end death, expresses the faith which 'makes them capable of being united in Christ with their loved ones who have already died, and gives them hope that they have found true life with God.[12]

The initial intercession of the Embolism is an immediate repetition of the final petition of the Our Father. Indeed, as Joseph Ratzinger (Pope Emeritus Benedict XVI) states, 'throughout the ages men and

---

9   John Navone, *Themes of St. Luke* (Rome: Gregorian University Press, 1970), 147.
10 Doireann Ní-Bhriain, *The Irish Times*, 16 June 2020.
11 *The Church in the Modern World*, 18, in Austin Flannery, ed., *Vatican Council II – The Basic Sixteen Documents* (Dublin: Dominican Publications, 2007).
12 Ibid.

women have interpreted this petition in a broader sense. In the midst of the world's tribulations they have also begged God to set a limit to the evils that ravage the world and our lives'.[13] The extension to engage 'every evil', expanding the concern of the Church to embrace the ills and injustices experienced in earthly existence, is fittingly expressed by Pope Benedict XVI: 'Yes, we may and we should ask the Lord also to free the world, ourselves, and the many individuals and peoples who suffer from the tribulations that make life almost unbearable'.[14]

Graciously grant peace in our days
The second element exchanges the positive for the negative, interceding for God to graciously grant the gift of peace, which will be repeated almost immediately in the *Prayer for Peace*. Noting that 'our word peace does not bring out all the richness of the Hebrew word *shalom* stem[ming] from a root which means to be whole, intact, finished, complete', Gisbert Ghysens states that it 'refers, of course, to individual happiness; but also (and more often) it looks to the collective prosperity of the nation as a whole'.[15] Like the biblical concept of justice, peace is a relational reality rooted in and resulting from the covenant with God. Peace is mentioned at the end of the beautiful blessing in the Book of Numbers, 'May the Lord bless you and keep you. May the Lord let his face shine on you and be gracious to you. May the Lord uncover his face and bring you peace' (Num 6:24–26). Indeed, this blessing bears the peace which many of the Psalms proclaim as the sign of God's presence. The fulfilment of God's faithfulness is often interpreted and indicated by the prophets in the bestowing of the Messianic blessing of peace. Some of the most powerful Old Testament texts in the Advent liturgy are assurances of peace in prosperity. Isaiah, in particular, points to the personification

13 Joseph Ratzinger, *Jesus of Nazareth: From the Baptism in the Jordan to the Transfiguration* (London: Bloomsbury, 2007), 167.
14 Ibid., 168.
15 Gisbert Ghysens, 'He Himself Is Our Peace', in Joseph A. Grispino, S.M., ed., *Foundations of Biblical Spirituality*, (London: Sands, 1964) 119-126, here 119.

in the Messianic prophecy: 'For there is a child born for us…and this is the name they give him… Prince-of-Peace' (Is 9:5).

In the New Testament Luke, seeing peace as a symbol of salvation, has Zechariah, the father of John the Baptist, point to the light of dawn that, delivering from 'darkness and the shadow of death', leads 'into the way of peace' (1:79). This sense of fulfilment is immediately felt by Simeon who declares that he is ready to depart in peace having seen the Messiah in the child Jesus in the Temple (2:29–32). Luke is the evangelist of peace, bracketing the ministry of Jesus between the announcement by the angels of the advent of peace and the announcement of the Risen Lord at his appearance to the anguished disciples, 'Peace be with you' (2:14; 24:36). As the apostle of peace Paul announces that Christ has come to proclaim 'peace to you who were far off and peace to those who were near, for through him both of us have access in one Spirit to the Father' (Eph 2:17–18). Paul presents peace positively, not purely as the end of hostility but as the experience of happiness that ends in holiness.

In the 'Farewell Discourse' of the Gospel of John, Jesus promises peace to his disciples. Chapter 14 begins with Jesus telling the disciples 'Do not let your hearts be troubled', which he doubles on with the addition 'and do not let them be afraid' (14:27). Between reassurance and repetition rests the revelation of peace: 'Peace I leave with you; my peace I give to you. I do not give as the world gives' (14:27). C. L. Mitton distinguishes three meanings of peace in the New Testament: peace as the opposite of conflict through the reconciliation between peoples realised in Christ, restoration of right relationship with God resulting in a state of righteousness, and 'peace of mind or serenity'.[16] Noting that the third of these 'appears to be a distinctively Christian meaning', he states that this spiritual sense, which subsumes both mind and heart, should be applied 'to John 14:27, since the gift of peace is explicitly offered in contrast to the troubled and fearful hearts of the disciples'.[17]

---

16 C. L. Mitton, 'Peace in the NT', in *The Interpreter's Dictionary of the Bible, K-Q*, (Nashville: Abingdon, 1962), 706.
17 Ibid.

The Embolism's inclusion of 'in our days' joins a sense of priority to both present protection and the rolling-out of a vaccine as a permanent prophylaxis in the future. This is now added to an already long list of prayer(s) for peace, ranging from regional conflicts with the potential of global repercussions through nuclear arms proliferation to the threat of environmental destruction. Cardinal Peter Turkson has identified how the COVID-19 pandemic is part of the overall problem and potential of peace: 'As the world takes emergency measures to address a global pandemic and a global economic recession, both underpinned by a global climate emergency, we must also consider the implications for peace of these interconnected crises'.[18]

By the help of your mercy

'O God, come to our aid / O Lord, make haste to help us' is the 'Introduction to Each Hour' in the daily *Divine Office* of the Church. This regular and general prayer for divine assistance is repeated in the third petition, specifically asking for the help of God's mercy. In recent times the theme of mercy has emerged prominently in the life of 'prayer and faith' within the Church. Building on Pope John Paul II's 1980 encyclical *Dives in Misericordia (Rich in Mercy)*, Pope Francis begins his document introducing the Extraordinary Year of Mercy, declaring, 'Jesus Christ is the face of the Father's mercy'.[19] His statement that 'these words might well sum up the mystery of the Christian faith' suggests the symbol of a horizon, an image specially favoured by him. The mercy which 'has become living and visible in Jesus of Nazareth, reaching its culmination in him' is the horizon within which God operates, outreaching to humanity and offering his mercy without reservation. This focus on mercy forms a vital resource for the Church in understanding and undertaking its ministry *ad intra* and its mission *ad extra*.

Luke is the evangelist who especially expounds that Jesus is the

---

18 'To prepare the future, to construct the peace in the time of COVID-19', Vatican Press Conference, 7 July 2020. https://press.vatican.va/content/salastampa/en/bollettino/pubblico/2020/07/07/200707a.html

19 Pope Francis, *Misericordiae Vultus* (Dublin: Veritas, 2015), 1.

pre-eminent expression and embodiment of God's mercy. He presents Jesus' injunction in Matthew 'to be perfect as your heavenly Father is perfect' (5:48) as the invitation in Luke to 'be merciful, just as your Father is merciful' (6:36). Portraying Jesus as the Messiah of God's mercy, who communicates and conducts himself as the compassionate Christ, Luke depicts how in word and deed, miracles and parables, he shows the merciful face of the Father, especially to the poor and the lost. The praying of Luke's *Benedictus* in the morning and *Magnificat* in the evening permits the Church to live 'by the tender mercy of our God' and 'in remembrance of his mercy'. Also, Luke alone presents the parables of pity, particularly that of the compassionate Samaritan. William Spohn's contrast between the two who saw the man left 'half dead' and passed by on the other side and the Samaritan, communicates the human face of mercy: 'The Samaritan sees the man as a fellow human being in terrible trouble...The priest and the Levite did not let themselves be affected by his plight... The Samaritan has no such emotional immunity.'[20] The example of the Samaritan, in the words of Carl R. Holladay about the Gospel of Luke, 'practicing uncalculating mercy',[21] ends with the exhortation of Jesus, 'Go and do likewise' (10:37).

Through plagues and other natural disasters, war and injustice, illness and death, the Bible portrays the mercy of God often coming to the help of suffering humanity. Prayer to God to continue to bestow his merciful help is a perennial feature of human experience, to which the present sad pandemic proves no exception.

That we may be always free from sin and safe from all distress
While the first petition prayed for deliverance 'from every evil', the fourth points particularly to two forms of evil, the one moral or theological, the other psychospiritual. Among the metaphors for thinking and talking theologically about sin 'which may speak

---

20   William Spohn, *Go and Do Likewise* (New York, Continuum, 1999), 89–90.
21   Carl R. Holladay, *A Critical Introduction to the New Testament – Interpreting the Message and Meaning of Jesus Christ* (Nashville: Abingdon Press, 2009), 181.

effectively to people today', Kenneth R. Himes selects that of sin as a virus.[22] A virus is a foreign body that enters the host entity and engenders a cycle of destruction which can end in its expiry. Himes interprets the image in medical terms, talking of 'the pathological [which] is like a cancer that grows and develops'.[23] While the image of sin as a virus is helpful in interpreting its effects, a downside is its impersonal nature and the danger of downplaying responsibility for the damage that is done even to the point of destruction and death. Government and public campaigns to counter the contagion of the coronavirus have emphasised the importance of individual responsibility in the context of social solidarity.

Affirming that 'to present the moral life in general and also that of the Christian in terms of an *ethic of responsibility* is an illuminating but also a challenging approach', Bill Cosgrave argues that 'it calls all of us, individuals, groups and communities, to examine our way of living and as moral people to assess our responsibility for the effects of our activity on the quality of life in our societies, especially on those who are poor'.[24] The relevance of this responsibility to root out coronavirus is a reminder to the Christian faithful of the need to call on the assistance of God to help in defeating not only the effects of the pandemic but also to deny any sinful attitudes or actions which could contribute to its continuation. The desire to be 'always free from sin' dovetails the human drive to goodness and the divine draw to holiness in the dialogue of freedom and grace.

Stay safe has been the public health message here since the lifting of lockdown. Posted on multiple television channels and other media platforms, it is a simple though not simplistic message, meant to stay the course of the COVID-19 crisis. Alongside disease, distress levels have deepened, giving rise to commentary and concern for mental health issues throughout society. Keeping the 'all' from a previous

---

22 Kenneth R. Himes, 'Human Failing: The Meanings and Metaphors of Sin' in James Keating, ed., *Moral Theology – New Directions and Fundamental Issues* (New York: Paulist Press, 2004), 145-161.

23 Ibid., 156.

24 Bill Cosgrave, 'Responsibility in the Christian Life', *The Furrow*, 71 (July/August 2020), 411--422, here 422.

translation, 'protect us from all anxiety', this petition is universal in both its appeal and agenda. The present focus on health and safety fits in with the desire for protection from distress and the many forms it assumes in human experience. While complete immunity from suffering is impossible, an illusion in the limited conditions of life, the intercession for 'safety from all distress' is identifiable as a human response to danger in all its dimensions.

The Psalms offer a rich resource for individual and communal prayer. Personal plight is presented profoundly in the lines 'I tell [the Lord] all my distress/for I am in the depths of distress' as the depth of desolation depicted here depends solely on the safety that God can send, 'You are my refuge, all I have left in the land of the living' (142[141]:3, 6–7). The affirmation in another Psalm, 'God is for us a refuge and strength, a helper close at hand, in time of distress' (46[45]:1), offers both a recognition of plight and a realisation of God's protective presence. Luke's depiction of the agony of Jesus in Gethsemane – 'In his anguish he prayed more earnestly, and his sweat became like great drops of blood falling down on the ground' (22:44) – describes the depths of distress to which Jesus descends.

Paul is the apostle of affliction, for as Frank J. Matera notes, 'these afflictions encompass the physical suffering and mental anguish that he endures because of his apostolic ministry'.[25] However, these hardships only serve to show the help with which 'the Father of mercies and the God of all consolation consoles us in all our affliction' (2 Cor 1:3–4). Furthermore, this is 'so that we may be able to console those who are in any affliction with the consolation with which we ourselves are consoled by God' (1:4). Both realistic and remarkable, this passage reminds us that while we may not be shielded from suffering, God will send safety which is often shown and seen in solidarity with and for the distressed. The final petition, 'safe from all distress', finishes the prayer for deliverance 'from every evil'.

---

25   Frank J. Matera, *II Corinthians – A Commentary* (Louisville: Westminster John Knox Press, 2003) 41.

Healing and Hope

The Embolism ends with a shift from asking to announcing, 'as we await the blessed hope and the coming of our Saviour, Jesus Christ'. Remembering that the Latin root of salvation is *salus*, health / safety / deliverance, this proclamation places all the previous petitions in an eschatological perspective, focussed on the person of Christ and his Second Coming. The hope heralded here is revealed, as in the words of Graham Ward: 'religious hope is indestructible. It is a hope beyond all human hoping… a blind hoping because we and the cultures we inhabit and shape are not its author and therefore do not control its operations, its secret workings within the heart of things human and nonhuman'.[26] It is *blessed hope* because 'since we have a great priest over the house of God, let us approach with a true heart in full assurance of faith' (Heb 10:21–22). The absolute assurance of faith is founded on the Resurrection, as articulated by Joseph Ratzinger: 'Hence in the extraordinary promise of this event there is also found an extraordinary call, a vocation, a whole interpretation of human existence and the existence of the world…Quite definitely, this is what faith in the Resurrection is concerned with: the real power of God, and the purport of human responsibility'.[27]

The pandemic has been a paschal experience for the Christian faithful who, 'made a partner in the paschal mystery and configured to the death of Christ, will go forward, strengthened by hope, to the resurrection'.[28] Christian hope is the hinge that holds together the human desire for happiness on earth and the divine draw to life in heaven. Even as the door of earthly existence closes, life does not end but opens into the eternal embrace of God. This opening enables, in the words of the Vatican International Theological Commission, 'the removal of the obstacles lying between God and us, and the offer to us of participating in God's life'.[29] Asking for healing here and

---

26 Graham Ward, 'Christian Hope Facing Secular Fatalism', *Doctrine & Life*, 70 (April 2020), 2–16, here 14.
27 Joseph Ratzinger, *Journey Towards Easter* (Slough: St Paul Publications, 1987), 116–117.
28 Vatican II, *The Church in the Modern World*, 22.
29 International Theological Commission, 'Select Questions on the Theology of God the Redeemer', *Communio* 24 (Spring 1977), 161, par 1.

now and announcing the hope of heaven, the *Embolism* entwines the earthly and eternal elements of existence. To adapt the subtitle of Butler's *Prayer*, this is the Christian adventure in living.

Questions for Reflection and Discussion

1. How, in the absence of social celebration and sacramental reception of the Eucharist, can the prayers of the Mass – especially the Embolism – help you grow spiritually through the COVID-19 crisis?

2. 'Peace of mind' is a phrase heard many times in relation to COVID-19. Reflect and share on the promise of Paul, 'And the peace of God, which surpasses all understanding, will guard your hearts and minds in Christ Jesus' (Phil 4:7).

3. Do you have a particular psalm that you pray 'in time of distress'?

4. The creed tells us: 'He will come again in glory to judge the living and the dead'. How does this profession of faith parallel praying the Embolism after the Our Father, particularly in a time of pandemic?

5. You are invited to pray this prayer (composed by author): 'God, our heavenly Father, grant us the fortitude of Christ your Son to face the COVID-19 crisis with trust, patience and compassion. Give us the grace of the Holy Spirit to free us from fear and look forward together to the future with healing and hope. Through the intercession of Saint Joseph, the guardian of Jesus, and Mary his mother and mother of the Church, may we be guided through this time of peril. Preserve us in peace; protect the vulnerable; keep safe our health care workers and all who serve society, at home and abroad. We ask this through Christ our Lord. Amen'.

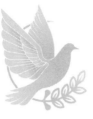

The 'Foolishness of the Daily' in Light of COVID-19: Reflections Towards a Christian Metaphysics

Philip John Paul Gonzales

The daily rhythm of our lives was interrupted in an unimaginable way with the appearance of COVID-19 onto the world-stage in 2020. Indeed, not since the Second World War have generations experienced such world-historical uncertainty, at least in western countries. This is not to say that COVID-19 is anywhere close to matching the horror and tragedy of that war, but it is to say that the level of uncertainty and disruption is dangerous and tangible. As time went on, we had an increasing number of questions: When will the pandemic end? Will we have to live with this virus forever, as some have suggested? Will a viable and effective vaccine be found, and if so, when? Are we at the beginning of this crisis, the midpoint or end? Will nationwide lockdowns be reinforced? What is going to happen to our late-Capitalist 'throw-away' (Pope Francis) global economy which has never been more interdependent? Will it merely contract, will it crash, will it recover or morph into something new?

On a deeply human level what is to happen to our human community – a community that cannot exist without the proximity of bodies? When will the smile of the human face be freed from the anonymity and faceless veil of medical masks? When will we be able to greet each other again with a kiss on the cheek or a shake of hands, for is it not these embodied gestures which build human community in the first place? When will pubs, those places of fellowship, be safe to return to? And, most importantly of all, when will the Eucharist return to us without the ever-present threat of new closures, or restrictions, of our churches? No one – and I mean no one – has been able to answer these questions with certainty!

What then are we Christians to do in the face of these overwhelming circumstances and extreme uncertainty? Before these world-historical powers it seems almost impossible not to feel helpless, insignificant and powerless. However, in the face of the COVID-19 crisis we must beware of that ever-present temptation of Christian life, namely, to become distracted by worries that remove our eyes from our vocation and work, along with daily crosses and vicissitudes that inevitably ensue. The paradigmatic warning against such a mind-set is expressed in Paul's writings to the Thessalonian community; a community that is largely overwhelmed by the imminent expectation of the Parousia or the Second Coming of Christ. This imminent expectation led many to adopt an attitude of indifference, inactivity and idleness before the cares and crosses of the daily life. Paul moves against this attitude with an exhortation of Christians to avoid neglecting these realities, cares and concerns of the daily Christian life. Present then in Paul's response to the Thessalonian community, in face of the ever-present possibility of the Apocalypse, is contained that kernel and unsurpassable treasure of Christian spirituality which I call the 'foolishness of the daily'. All orthodox Christian spiritualities are grounded in the 'foolishness of the daily'.

This foolishness was inaugurated in the radical veiled lowliness of the mother of God, shared with the kenotic (self-emptying) hidden life of the Word made flesh before his public manifestation. It is seen in the great rule of Benedict and its attention to the minutiae of the daily. It is there in St Francis's rule which is tied so closely to a form of life, as well as his belief that the greatest manner of preaching is via action and an embodied faith and life rather than via words. It is there in the hagiographic anecdote of the life of Bonaventure who, it is said, was washing dishes when presented with the cardinal's hat, to which he responded, put it out on that tree and I will get it when I am finished with the dishes. It is there in the great mystic Teresa of Avila's famed statement that God is found in the pots and the pans. It is there in the Ignatian spirituality of finding God in all things (the concrete and history). It is there in the 'little way' of Thérèse of Lisieux, which teaches that the smallest action done with great love is a world-altering event. It is there in the life and witness of Maximilian Kolbe before and within Auschwitz. These saints are just some of the countless examples offered from the living mosaic of Christian life and spirituality. This 'foolishness of the daily' teaches the deepest Christian truth that those that are not faithful in the little things will fail at great things when, and if, the time presents itself.

In a poignant way, the 'foolishness of the daily' is there in the 'hidden life' of Franz Jägerstätter, and his wife Franziska, along with their three daughters.[1] The daily spiritual drama unfolded with Franz's grace-filled sacrifice in having to give up his life – and life must here be understood as his shared life with his wife and children – because of his refusal to serve in Hitler's army despite the pressure of his village, and tragically, the Catholic prelates. The meaning of the 'foolishness of the daily' became evident in the rhythm of the daily realities of an Austrian farmer and the common life of his family amidst the impending apocalyptic destruction unleashed in the political ideology of National Socialism. This is thus an eschatological confrontation between the humble and loving acts of daily life, and their seeming insignificance, in the face of overwhelming political power and darkness that is enveloping everything. It is the true story

---

1   See Franz Jägerstätter, *Franz Jägerstätter: Letters and Writings from Prison*, trans. Robert A. Krieg, ed. Erna Putz (Maryknoll, NY: Orbis Books, 2009). The phrase 'hidden life', in this context, is taken from the deeply haunting and poetic depiction of the life of Jägerstätter in Terrence Malick's recent film *A Hidden Life* (2019). This is not to say that the film fully captures – as this is an impossibility – the daily drama of Franz's sacrifice of his life.

of the hidden powerless power of kenotic love in daily life lived in resistance to God-less power and control. Likewise, it is no felicitous accident that Maximilian Kolbe gave his life, as a priest and friar, in substitution of a young father of a family – thus giving back to this young father the gift of the daily in the common life with his family, a common life that was taken from Franz. One sacrifice comes out of the 'foolishness of the daily,' while the other returns life to the 'foolishness of the daily': the heart of Christian life.

The great disciples of the 'foolishness of the daily' lived and performed a metaphysics of action – or better, what Balthasar called a 'metaphysics of the saints'.[2] Today we rarely think of metaphysics and spirituality as being linked, and this is one of the direst effects that modernity has had upon the fullness of Christian vision, where its mosaic has become compartmentalised and fractured. However, in the greatest Christian minds, spirituality and deep metaphysical and theological realities of the Christian faith were always intertwined. Let me all-too-briefly explain how a 'metaphysics of the saints' is closely aligned to a spirituality of the 'foolishness of the daily'. Christian metaphysics is rooted in the mysterious reality of God's love expressed in the gift of creation (and re-creation, as will be seen). In this view God freely creates without the slightest bit of necessity to do so. Hence, creation is what is freely given as what is other to God himself. In common parlance, if something that does not need to be given is given freely, we call what is given a *gift*. If one is forced to give something, it is not a gift. Moreover, in a common understanding of a gift, one is able to distinguish the giver from the gift. The gift is not the giver and nor is the giver the gift.

God's gift of creation is not God and God is not creation. But because creation is a gift it bespeaks the presence of the giver. The response to the gift and the presence of the giver in the gift is gratitude and thankfulness. Christian metaphysics is thus rooted in the

2   For this beautiful phrase see Hans Urs von Balthasar, *The Glory of the Lord: A Theological Aesthetics*, vol. V: *The Realm of Metaphysics in the Modern Age,* trans. Oliver Davies et al. (San Francisco: Ignatius Press, 1991), 48–140.

fundamental Christian truth that we were loved into being and thus we were loved before we ourselves ever loved. Christian metaphysics teaches humanity how to see and receive life and being as a gift, and thus to respond with gratitude and thanksgiving, that is *(eucharistia)* understood as thanksgiving. In other words, Christian metaphysics teaches the Christian what we are, namely, a creature of God and thus a gift which has been given. Response to this gift, in turn, demands gratitude and thanksgiving that knows it can never repay such a debt. Here we come to know ourselves in our absolute creaturely poverty.

A Christian metaphysics is a metaphysics of poverty and child-hood, where we learn to *receive* our fleshed and fragile creaturehood as it is, and thus as something that is always dependent on the Christian God. This kind of metaphysics seeks to enact this thanksgiving in the creaturehood and humanness of our fragile flesh. It is not just a thought or a concept but a life that seeks to live in response to the gift of life and being. In a word, it is also (and at the same time) a spirituality and this, in a nutshell, is what is meant by a 'metaphysics of the saints'. The saints, then, are those that live most deeply a life of thanksgiving and thankfulness in response to the reception of being as a gift and our recreation offered in Christ's redemptive work. The saints are those that enter most deeply into the mystery of our humanity in relation to its utter dependence on God. This means that, in practice, God is glorified most in the humble drudgery and vicissitudes of daily life – the wakening up every day to the same humble tasks and difficulties, and the crosses of the daily life.

When life and being are not seen as a gift, such daily cares and sufferings are nothing more than monotonous drudgery devoid of meaning and purpose; a prison routine without escape or joy. But the saint is the one who unlocks and unleashes the foolish, humble, childlike wisdom of the ordinary and daily, thereby seeing the extraor-dinary in the ordinary. Here the daily toil, drudgery and exhaustion are transmuted into the eucharistic thanksgiving of service. The pain of self-gift and self-giving is a life of service lived, in joy, for others in the daily cares of life as the only place wherein our thanksgiving can truly be made and offered. Christian metaphysics and spirituality always coalesce in an incarnation of gratitude in response to the two-fold gift of love as seen in humanity's creation and redemption. But such an incarnation must, of necessity, occur within the horizon of the ordinary and daily realities of life. This is the wisdom of the cross, seen in a life given over to the foolish hiddenness of the daily.

We can wax lyrical about the adventure of Christian sanctity, we can be filled with the fire of this love because, as Léon Bloy saw, the only tragedy in life is not becoming a saint.[3] Yet, we must abandon a hagiography of angelism, where saints are portrayed as haloed and crowned throughout their life and thus hardly human. Saints are human, indeed all-too-human. And thus the wealth of sanctity is found in the poverty of the daily and their glory in the pain and exhaustion of service, as so masterfully portrayed in the character of M. le Curé in Bernanos's novel, *The Diary of a Country Priest*.[4] Failure and the overwhelming sense and feeling of failure are thus part and parcel of sanctity.

World-history and its great events of wealth, fame, victory and violent conquest march on; both indifferent and mocking of the foolish failure of sanctity's quotidian existence. Events forever out of our control, and spheres of influence beyond our reach, are ever happening. COVID-19 and its yet-to-be-known historical fallout is one of these events which bring us face-to-face with our own powerlessness in relation to events of global order. What are we to do when faced with our own powerlessness to control and influence a pandemic that is rapidly spreading around the world? The answer is the same as it always was, and always will be, from the time of Mary and Christ, to the Christian community of Thessalonica, to the great figures of Christian sanctity, until the Second Coming.

The answer is ever-ancient and ever-new: our strength lies in our weakness, our wealth in our poverty, our glory in the inglorious, as

---

3   See Léon Bloy, *The Woman who was Poor* (London: Sheed & Ward, 1939).
4   See Georges Bernanos, *The Diary of a Country Priest*, trans. Pamela Morris (Glasgow: Collins, 1981).

seen in the ever-demanding taking-up of the cross. Here we find the foolish wisdom of the daily, exhibited in the service of a Christian 'metaphysics of the saints', which ever lives out of a being – true to the truth that 'whoever would save his life will lose it: and whoever loses his life for my sake will find it' (Mt 16:25).[5]

Questions for Reflection and Discussion

1. Within our own lives, can we find value in the 'foolishness of the daily'?
2. If we think of canonised saints or good people we have known, which of them have shown us how to live amid the trials of this world?
3. Do we agree that, in practice, God is glorified most in the humble drudgery and vicissitudes of daily life?
4. When faced with our own powerlessness to control and influence the pandemic, can we accept that our strength actually lies in our weakness?

---

5   It is perhaps more than fitting that this sentence is followed by Christ alluding to his Second Coming. What should we do before this ever-present possibility of Christ's return? Simply take up our cross daily and follow him. The Christian life is the apocalyptic drama of the daily in its extreme urgency to respond to Christ's love in the now.

Frequently Cited Sources

Catechism of the Catholic Church (CCC), www.vatican.va/archive/ENG0015/_INDEX.HTM.

Pope Francis, *Evangelii Gaudium* (EG), www.vatican.va/content/francesco/en/apost_exhortations/documents/papa-francesco_esortazione-ap_20131124_evangelii-gaudium.html.

Pope Francis, *Fratelli Tutti* (FT), www.vatican.va/content/francesco/en/encyclicals/documents/papa-francesco_20201003_enciclica-fratelli-tutti.html.

Pope Francis, *Gaudete et Exsultate* (GE), www.vatican.va/content/francesco/en/apost_exhortations/documents/papa-francesco_esortazione-ap_20180319_gaudete-et-exsultate.html.

Irish Catholic Bishops' Conference, *Parish Pastoral Councils, a Framework for Developing Diocesan Norms and Parish Guidelines*, www.catholicbishops.ie/wp-content/uploads/images/stories/cco_publications/pastoralrenewal/pastoral_councils_book_final-1.pdf.

John Paul II, *Catechesi Tradendae* (CT), www.vatican.va/content/john-paul-ii/en/apost_exhortations/documents/hf_jp-ii_exh_16101979_catechesi-tradendae.html.

Archbishop Eamon Martin, *Homily for Ascension Sunday / World Communications Day*, www.catholicbishops.ie/2020/05/24/homily-of-archbishop-eamon-martin-for-ascension-sunday-world-communications-day.

Note from the Apostolic Penitentiary on the Sacrament of Reconciliation in the current pandemic, 20/03/2020, press.vatican.va/content/salastampa/en/bollettino/pubblico/2020/03/20/200320d.html.

Pontifical Council for Justice and Peace, *Compendium of the Social Doctrine of the Church* (CSDC), www.vatican.va/roman_curia/pontifical_councils/justpeace/documents/rc_pc_justpeace_doc_20060526_compendio-dott-soc_en.html.

Vatican II, *Gaudium et Spes* (GS), www.vatican.va/archive/hist_councils/ii_vatican_council/documents/vat-ii_cons_19651207_gaudium-et-spes_en.html.

Vatican II, *Lumen Gentium* (LG), www.vatican.va/archive/hist_councils/ii_vatican_council/documents/vat-ii_const_19641121_lumen-gentium_lt.html.

Vatican II, *Sacrosanctum Concilium* (SC), www.vatican.va/archive/hist_councils/ii_vatican_council/documents/vat-ii_const_19631204_sacrosanctum-concilium_en.html.

List of Contributors

Thomas G. Casey, SJ, Professor of Philosophy, St Patrick's College, Maynooth

Anne Codd, PBVM, Occasional Lecturer, Pastoral Theology, St Patrick's College, Maynooth

Pádraig Corkery, Lecturer in Moral Theology, St Patrick's College, Maynooth

Jeremy Corley, Lecturer in Sacred Scripture, St Patrick's College, Maynooth

Philip John Paul Gonzales, Lecturer in Philosophy, St Patrick's College, Maynooth

Michael Hurley, Parish Priest of Bohernabreena, Co. Dublin

Austen Ivereigh, Fellow in Contemporary Church History, Campion Hall, Oxford University

Gaven Kerr, Lecturer in Philosophy, St Patrick's College, Maynooth

Nóirin Lynch, Director of Margaret Aylward Centre, Glasnevin, Dublin

Eamon Martin, Archbishop of Armagh, Chancellor of St Patrick's College, Maynooth

Aoife McGrath, Director of Pastoral Theology, St Patrick's College, Maynooth

Michael Mullaney, President, St Patrick's College, Maynooth

Neil Xavier O'Donoghue, Lecturer in Systematic Theology, St Patrick's College, Maynooth

Kevin O'Gorman, SMA, Lecturer in Moral Theology, St Patrick's College, Maynooth

Noel O'Sullivan, Lecturer in Systematic Theology, St Patrick's College, Maynooth

Jessie Rogers, Lecturer in Sacred Scripture, St Patrick's College, Maynooth

Salvador Ryan, Professor of Ecclesiastical History, St Patrick's College, Maynooth

John-Paul Sheridan, Director of Education Programmes, St Patrick's College, Maynooth

Michael Shortall, Lecturer in Moral Theology, St Patrick's College, Maynooth

Select Index